Public Education about Cancer

UICC Monograph Series · Volume 5

Public Education about Cancer

Research findings and theoretical concepts

Prepared by the Committee on Public Education
of the Commission on Cancer Control

Research and background material by Michael S. Goodstadt

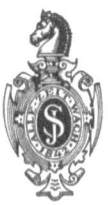

Springer-Verlag Berlin Heidelberg GmbH

ISBN 978-3-642-88008-7   ISBN 978-3-642-88006-3 (eBook)
DOI 10.1007/978-3-642-88006-3
Originally published by Springer-Verlag Berlin Heidelberg in 1967
Softcover reprint of the hardcover 1st edition 1967

Library of Congress Catalog Card Number 66-29 248

Title-No. 7516

Preface

This monograph is essentially the outcome of corporate endeavour on the part of members of the Committee on Public Education of the International Union against Cancer, from the decision taken in September 1963, via a lengthy and arduous reworking of the first draft in Philadelphia in 1964 to its final editorial meeting in September 1965. In between there has been a continuous exchange of ideas, suggestions, advice and material for inclusion. Nevertheless, as chairman I should be remiss if I did not acknowledge the Committee's indebtedness to Mr. MICHAEL S. GOODSTADT, formerly of the University of Manchester, who worked with me in Manchester and undertook the painstaking search of sources of published information and compiled the draft on which this monograph is based. If there are omissions from the bibliography, it is not for want of industry in seeking them out: our difficulty has been to obtain original material from certain sources.

We hope that the material assembled here will both offer useful guidance to those engaged in public education about cancer and provide a baseline from which future research in this neglected field may stem.

Contents

Introduction
Public Education in Cancer Control

There has been an increasing realization in recent years that education of the public about cancer is an essential element of cancer control and prevention. In 1963 an Expert Comittee of the World Health Organization said in its report *Cancer Control:* "Health education of the population and of patients is an integral part of a cancer control programme and an essential element in the success of most control measures. Experience in many countries indicates that there is considerable public interest in the subject and widespread readiness to cooperate with the health authorities in the prevention, detection, diagnosis, treatment and after-care of cancer when the problems involved are properly understood". In 1964 another W. H. O. Expert Committee, reporting on *Prevention of Cancer,* reinforced these comments by its expressed belief that prevention is impossible without education. The report continued "The combination of medical action and health education, which has been so effective in combating infectious and nutritional diseases, can now be applied in the field of cancer prevention." The Expert Committee also drew attention to a serious deficiency: "The educational problems of cancer prevention have not received as much attention as other aspects of cancer. There are wide gaps in our knowledge of social, psychological and educational factors that inhibit the utilization of preventive knowledge, and expenditure on research in health education concerning cancer is negligible."

While it is true that research of this kind is still woefully inadequate, there is a considerable body of useful material available; but much of it has appeared in journals that are either not readily accessible, or unfamiliar, to workers in the field of cancer. For this reason, the Committee on Public Education of the U.I.C.C. decided at its meeting in Geneva, 19—20 September 1963, to undertake the compilation of a Monograph which would bring together in convenient form some of the more important studies relating to public education.

Many of the publications discussed or listed in this monograph are concerned directly with aspects of the cancer problem. Others bear either on the general principles of health education and behavioural change, or on the similar difficulties encountered in other health problems in which fear, emotion and prejudice play a large part. There are, for example, several parallels to be drawn between public attitudes to mental health and to cancer.

It would be convenient if public education about cancer could be reduced to some simple formula that would fit all countries. Unfortunately, no such easy solution is possible. As in all forms of health education, a number of general principles can be formulated, but how they are put into practice must always depend on local beliefs, conditions and resources. It would be pointless, for example, to make generalizations about the use of newspaper publicity, since the distribution of newspapers and the degree of literacy in the population varies so much from country to country. Every medium of publicity can be employed, from the large-scale use of newspapers, films, radio and television to the more personal forms of persuasion exercised by doctors on their patients. There is no special magic in any one medium of publicity: it cannot be said that lectures are better than films, or that pamphlets are better than posters. All can play their part in informing the public, but these are merely the tools of the health educator. Their effectiveness lies solely in the skill and aptness with which they are applied to the problems to be solved.

The main purpose of this Monograph is to make available, particularly to those whose initial training has been in other fields, an introduction to the considerable body of published knowledge available from the disciplines now commonly grouped under the heading 'behavioural studies', i.e. psychology, sociology, social anthropology and educational theory. We cannot hope to present all these findings in concise form, but we have tried to direct workers in the field of public education about cancer to some of the most interesting and profitable sources of information basic to their craft. This publication therefore takes the form of an extensive annotated bibliography rather than a self-sufficient text. While so many gaps remain in our knowledge, some of the findings are contradictory. Often the ideal situation visualized by the researchers has to give way to expediency, and sensible compromise becomes necessary. Nevertheless, for all their shortcomings, these findings are stimulating and cannot be ignored.

In view of the immense current interest in the subject, readers may be surprised to find no detailed treatment of research into ways of changing smoking habits, particularly in the young. This omission is not because the subject was not considered important, but because we felt that it could not be treated adequately within the framework of the present monograph. The Committee has already decided that a further report devoted solely to health education and tobacco smoking should be prepared as its next major undertaking.

In introducing this report, the Committee wishes to put on record its deep conviction that education of the general public is vital if the full potential of our present preventive measures, diagnostic tools and treatment methods is ever to be achieved. Prompt treatment for cancer is essential, and as long as people delay before seeking a doctor's advice for symptoms which may be caused by cancer, thousands of needless deaths — estimated at about 92,000 annually in the U.S.A. alone — will continue to occur. People cannot act in the ways most likely to help them if they are either ignorant of the facts, or afflicted by a paralysing fear of cancer. Public education, using whatever resources are available locally, has the task of creating a climate of acceptance of the benefits of seeking medical advice promptly. It must encourage a rational view of cancer as a group of diseases, many forms of which are highly curable if treated at an early stage, even though other forms remain difficult to treat successfully. It may also, as has happened in the past, provide an effective spur to official action or to the moulding of medical opinion.

But these are secondary though welcome by-products of educating the public. The main aim, in simple words, is to reassure people and to teach them to act appropriately, to reduce cancer in the public mind from its present fearful eminence to the level of other serious but controllable diseases.

References

Cancer Control, *Wld. Hlth. Org. techn. Rep. Ser. 251* (1963).

Prevention of Cancer, *Wld. Hlth. Org. techn. Rep. Ser., 276* (1964).

Section I

Attitudes to Cancer

1. The Nature of Attitudes to Cancer and General Medical Practices

This chapter will deal with topics related directly to attitudes to cancer and other diseases; the nature, sources, and extent of these attitudes both in the medical profession and in the general population.

A number of studies have been concerned with the nature of attitudes to disease, but for obvious reasons, priority is given here to those attitudes concerned with cancer. To forestall any objections that the meaning of the term "attitude" has not been clarified, let it be said here that we have thought it preferable to leave such theoretical considerations until after the objective experimental results have been presented.

Few studies have been concerned solely with people's attitudes to cancer; those which do exist are concerned with evidence for or against the existence of widespread cancerophobia. However, indirect reference to and evidence about attitudes to cancer can be found in studies concerned with the public's state of knowledge, with reactions to having cancer and being told the diagnosis, and with delay in seeking medical care. Studies concerned with cancer education also throw some light on the subject. All these aspects will be discussed in detail later. More direct evidence is provided by LEVINE (1962) and NUNNALLY (1961), who found that cancer was rated highest in producing anxiety compared with other diseases.

References: Attitudes to cancer

DARGENT, M., (1962). La cancérophobie. *Acta Un. int. Cancr.* 18, 709.
476 cases of cancerophobia, one third of which were neurotic, two-thirds had a normal fear. Only 3.5 % of the 476 in fact had a neoplasm.

DARGENT, M., and VAUTERIN, C. (1961). La cancérophobie. *Sem. Hôp. Paris.* 37, 2417.

DONALDSON, M. (1955). Cancer: The psychological disease. *Lancet* i, 959 and later correspondence.

DONALDSON, M. (1958). Early diagnosis of cancer. A psychological problem. *Lancet* ii, 790.
"Although true cancerophobia is rare, both personal apprehension (which can be prevented by education) and impersonal cancer apprehension ('fear of creating fear') are almost universal."

LEVINE, G. N. (1962). Anxiety about illness: Psychological and social bases. *J. Hlth hum. Behav.* 3, 30.
National sample of 2970. Cancer more feared than polio, cerebral palsy, arthritis, birth defects and T. B. Positively correlated with fear of cancer were the factors: knowing a victim, knowledge about the disease, perceived prevalence, perceived expensiveness of treatment. Negatively correlated with fear of cancer are education and possession of adequate community medical resources.

NUNNALLY jr., J. C. (1961). *Popular conceptions of mental health: Their development and change*, New York: Holt, Rinehart & Winston, Inc., p. 62.
Incidental to the author's examination of attitudes to mental health, he found that methods for treating cancer aroused the most anxiety when compared with meth-

ods for treating broken bones and mental illness.

SAMP, R. J. (1962). Physician poll on cancer preventon. Opinions and reactions of over 1,400 Doctors. *J. Amer. med. Ass.* **179**, 1001.

Evidence that "generally the ideas of preventing cancer seem novel, ineffective, and speculative" to doctors.

THOMAS, A. (1952). Typical patient and family attitudes. *Publ. Hlth. Rep. Wash.)* **67**, 960.

The author highlights the psychosocial, informational and experiential factors in a person's reaction to terminal cancer. A person's attitude to cancer will, in turn, affect that of other patients and families.

WAKEFIELD, J., and DAVISON, R. L. (1958). An answer to some criticisms of cancer education: A survey among general practitioners. *Brit. med. J.* **i**, 96.

The Authors found no cancerophobia resulting from an intensive cancer education programme.

World Health Organization (1964). Prevention of cancer. *Wld. Hlth. Org. techn. Rep. Ser. 276.*

"The warnings that cancer education might create cancerophobia have proved a myth" (p. 31).

The Doctor Looks at the cancer program (1956). *J. Amer. med. Ass.* **160**, 1171.

An editorial review of a report of National Opinion Research Center interviews with 500 physicians, named by their patients as family doctors in an earlier random sample study of adult U.S. population. Study indicates that the "average physician strongly endorses the American Cancer Society's injunction to 'go straight to your doctor at the first sign' of any of the 'seven danger signals.'" Despite minority criticism, "great majority of practicing physicians in the United States regard the major voluntary health agencies as useful allies in the continuing fight against ignorance and disease."

Opinion surveys on cancer

A much richer source of information concerning attitudes to cancer is to be found in the several surveys which have specifically attempted to assess the state of knowledge among the general population. These surveys ask questions, some of which require factual answers and others which call for answers that are more often a statement of opinion than of fact. Some of the stated opinions border on expressions of attitude. It is these opinions, and the general correctness or otherwise of the public's knowledge, that are of great importance to the health educator, since ignorance of the facts cannot help in producing reasonable behaviour and will often hinder it. Even more serious is the possession of over-pessimistic information, for this will almost certainly be a barrier to acting in the way reasonably demanded by the situation. This is not to be confused with the kind of ignorance that is combined with awareness of that ignorance, which often leads, for example, to going to the doctor to be advised about unusual symptoms. Thus, without postulating that undesirable attitudes always underly faulty knowledge, it is clear that the resulting behaviour will often be the same in both cases.

The four major series of surveys reviewed and summarized in this section are from (1) Manchester, England (1954, 1958, 1964); (2) Canada (1955, 1961); (3) United States (1948 — summarized in the 1956 report, 1956, 1964). (4) Perth, Australia (1965). There are also surveys from Poland (1963), Argentina (1963) and Italy (1963), and a very interesting study from the U.S.A. reported by LEVINE (1962). The surveys discussed here are listed in detail at the end of this section. For convenience, they are referred to in the text merely by the place of origin. The dates quoted are the years of publication of the Survey findings, not the years in which the surveys were carried out.

1. The true position of cardiac and vascular diseases as the main cause of

death in the countries where the surveys were carried out (Manchester 1954; Canada 1955; see also CARTWRIGHT 1958) is not reflected in the replies to the question "which illness kills the most people in this country?" Canada (1961), and even more so Perth (1965), showed that people's knowledge concerning the mortality rates for the different diseases was more correct than that shown in earlier surveys.

2. Answers to other questions demonstrate the anxiety associated with cancer, and also the fact that correct knowledge is no guarantee of fear-free attitudes. Two-thirds to three-quarters of those interviewed think cancer is the most alarming or serious of several specified diseases (Manchester 1954, 1958, 1964; Canada 1955, 1961; Perth 1965; Argentina 1963); the same holds true in the Polish survey and in the one reported by LEVINE (1962).

3. People's opinions on the curability of cancer ought to reflect their general opinions on cancer. The results of this question show variations according to (a) country (b) year asked. In the latest Manchester interim survey (1964), there was a continuing tendency for the proportion of people who still regard cancer as wholly incurable to fall to the lower levels of the Canadian survey (about 30%). The percentage for Perth (1965) was 40%. Reviewing the American surveys HORN and WAINGROW (1964) report that whereas 25.8% in 1940 thought that cancer is always incurable only 73.5% did so in 1962. Interestingly, however, more people in Canada than in the U.S.A. thought that cancer is always or sometimes curable. In the Argentine survey 39%, and in the Italian 93.3% of the factory workers and 80.8% of the senior students regarded cancer as incurable. The phrasing of the question in the Italian survey may have accounted for

these extraordinarily high percentages. The form of the questions about curability differed slightly in the various surveys: they were as follows:

Canada, Manchester and Perth: "Can any of them (five listed diseases) be cured or not?"

United States: "Do you know whether there is anything the doctor can do to cure cancer?"

Argentina: "What possibilities of cure do you think exist?"

Italy: "Do you think a cancer patient:
a) can, if treated, be definitely cured?
b) can hope only for temporary relief?
c) will in any case die of cancer?"

4. Another important indication of the general climate of public opinion regarding cancer is the response to questions about the efficacy or otherwise of prompt treatment, that is, treatment begun as soon as possible after the patient has first noticed signs or symptoms. Again the level of hopeful opinion varies with the country and year.

The Manchester figures have shown an improvement from 57% to 70% and the Canadian from 80% to 87%, in the proportion who believe that early treatment increases the chance of cure; the figure of 68% in Perth is comparable. Yet this still leaves 10%—20% who think that early treatment does not help. The figures were similar in the Argentine survey, which also showed that men held this opinion more than women, but in the Italian survey only 45% of the factory workers believed that early treatment helps.

5. Questions regarding experience of cancer among those interviewed showed that in Manchester about three-quarters knew of a close friend or relative who had suffered from cancer; in America the figure was 50% in 1948 and 1956, and 62% in 1964. Levine (1962) concludes that "people who know a victim of a disease — particularly someone close to

them — are more likely to say they fear the maladies 'a lot' than those who do not know a victim". However, there were less than 30% in England and America, 37% in Perth, and 50% in Canada, who said they knew or had heard of someone being cured of cancer. The correlation between experience with cancer patients and fear of cancer, and belief in curability, was brought out much more clearly in the Argentine survey. It should be noted here that the lay conception of cure is difficult to define: in general it means being made better and having no further trouble from that particular disorder. Doctors accept this but require more precision for their professional discussion and statistical evaluations of treatment. They therefore use as their criterion the fact that a patient is alive and without evidence of the disease 5 years or more after treatment, so allowing for the possibility of recurrence in certain types of cancer.

6. In all surveys, questions were asked about the signs and symptoms of possible cancer. Although there were large variations between the surveys, three findings stand out: (a) most respondents knew the significance of a lump in the breast; (b) far fewer knew the significance of vaginal bleeding, or discharge after the change of life: (c) signs or symptoms affecting other parts of the body are relatively and often absolutely less well-known. LEVINE 1962 found that people who knew a cancer victim tended to regard themselves as knowledgeable about the disease.

7. Except in the Argentine survey, only a very small minority of those interviewed were wholly ignorant of the treatment for cancer (Manchester 1954, Canada 1961, America 1948, 1956, Perth 1965, Poland 1963).

8. In most of the surveys, questions were asked regarding the cause of cancer. Although there has been overall improve-

ment with time, and more people are aware of cigarette smoking as a cause of cancer, there are still large pockets of superstitious opinion.

About 25% still believe cancer is hereditary (8 surveys), 7—15% believe it to be contagious (8 surveys), 12—20% believe it to be connected with hygiene (4 surveys), and for 15—25% it has overtones of immorality (4 surveys). There is evidence that a considerable number of people still believe cancer can becaused by everyday knocks and bumps. (cf. also CARTWRIGHT and MARTIN, 1958; and TOCH et al., 1961).

9. In the 1961 Canadian and the two early American surveys, a question was asked about why people delay going to see the doctor if they suspect cancer. The results show that, of those who thought a person would delay, 70% believed they would do so because of fear. The deep-seated nature of fear of cancer is shown in the Manchester surveys (1954, 1958), in which the question was asked why women are more often frightened of getting cancer than, for example, heart trouble; nearly three-quarters of them expressed fatalism (40%), fear of pain (20—30%), unspecified fear (10%).

10. In two American surveys (HORN 1956), a question was put asking why people think *others* delay. To the question "If a person thought he might have cancer, would he go to the doctor right away, or would he wait?" The number who replied "Would wait" fell from 21% to 12% in the 7 years between the two surveys, though the answer "Go right away" remained almost constant at 69% and 70%.

11. In the 1954 Manchester survey and the two Canadian surveys, respondents were asked if there is anything a person can do to prevent himself getting cancer: about 60% said there is nothing one can do. In the 1964 Manchester sur-

vey, 50% held the same opinion about prevention of cancer of the womb. A national survey carried out in the U.S.A. in 1964 showed a marked improvement in knowledge and use of several cancer detection tests. The proportion of women in 1964 who had heard of the tests were as follows: chest x-ray 84%, skin examination 68%, proctoscopic examination 56%, breast examination 83%, Papanicolaou test 77%. For men the proportions were: chest x-ray 83%, skin 58%, and proctoscopic 46%. (American Cancer Society 1964). The Perth survey showed that though 80% of the respondents (male and female) had never had a cancer check-up, an even higher proportion were favourably disposed to such measures.

12. In all the surveys except those in Canada, a correlation was found between the state of knowledge or attitudes and the socio-economic level of the respondents. This finding is important, because for some forms of cancer those lowest on the socioeconomic scale constitute the high-risk groups (e. g. cancer of the uterine cervix).

References: Major public opinion surveys on cancer

(N.B. The dates refer to publication: in each instance the survey was carried out earlier.)

Argentina:

1964: SEEBER, A. B. de S., Public opinion on cancer in Argentina. *U.I.C.C. Bull.* 2, No. 4, 3, (1964).

Australia, Perth:

1965: *A social survey of community attitudes to cancer.* Cancer Council of Western Australia 1966.

Canada:

1955: PHILLIPS, A. J. Public opinion on cancer. *Canad. med. Ass. J.* 73, 639, (1955).

1961: PHILLIPS, A. J., and TAYLOR, R. M. Public opinion on cancer in Canada: A second survey. *Canad. med. Ass. J.* 84, 142 (1961).

England, Manchester:

1954: PATERSON, R., and AITKEN-SWAN, J. Public opinion on cancer: A survey among women in The Manchester Area. *Lancet* ii, 857, (1954).

1958: PATERSON, R., and AITKEN-SWAN, J. Public opinion on cancer: Changes following five years of cancer education. *Lancet* ii, 791, (1958).

1964: *Women's knowledge of and opinions on cancer.* An Interim Pilot Survey for the Manchester Comittee on Cancer (Manchester: Derek Roe Associates Ltd.)

Italy:

1963: MORANDI, G., VIVORI, C. e MENGON, M., Le conoscenze e gli orientamenti del pubblico in tema di tumori maligni [Public opinion and knowledge about cancer]. *Riv. med. Trentina 1,* 69, (1963). (Italian text.)

Poland:

1963: SAWICKI, F. Opinia publiczna o nowotworach [Public opinion about neoplastic diseases]. *Zdrow. publ.* 12, 599, (1963). (Russian and English Summaries.)

United States of America:

1948: Summarized in 1956 and 1964 (below).

1956: HORN, D. *et al.* Public opinion on cancer and the American Cancer Society: A report of a national Sample Survey. New York: American Cancer Society Inc. 1956.

1964: HORN, D., and WAINGROW, S. What changes are occuring in public opinion toward cancer: National public opinion survey. *Amer. J. publ. Hlth.* 54, 431, (1964).

Other references

Amer. Cancer Soc. (1964). *The public's awareness and use of cancer detection tests.* A Survey for the American Cancer Society. (Gallup Organization, Inc. Princeton, New Jersey.)

CARTWRIGHT, A., and MARTIN, F. M. (1958). Some popular beliefs concerning the causes of cancer. *Brit. Med. J.* ii, 592.

CARTWRIGHT, A., MARTIN, F. M., and THOMSON, J. G. (1958). Public opinion concerning tuberculosis. *Med. Off.* 99, 73.

KEGELES, S. S., KIRSCHT, J. P., HAEFNER, D. P., and ROSENSTOCK, I. M. (1965). Survey of beliefs about cancer detection and taking Papanicolaou tests. *Publ. Hlth. Rep.* 80, 815.

Behavioural scientists at the University of Michigan School of Public Health, analysing a national probability sample of whom 884 were women, confirm earlier reports that low socio-economic groups and women over 65 are least informed of the value of cervical tests. Those who know the benefits of tests tend to have them more regularly. The authors feel tests should be the subject of education at the time when women visit physicians and clinics. Physicians must explain to women the importance of these tests as they give them and must emphasize the benefits of early diagnosis. A greater mass information effort is needed.

LEVINE, G. N. (1962). Anxiety about Illness: Psychological and social bases. *J. Hlth. hum. Behav.* 3, 30.

TOCH, H., ALLEN, T., and LAZER, W. (1961). The public image of cancer etiology. *Public Opinion Quarterly* 25, 411.

WAKEFIELD, J., and BARIC, L. (1965). Public and professional attitudes to a screening programme for the prevention of cancer of the uterine cervix. *Brit. J. prev. soc. Med.* 19, 151.

Other studies

In addition to the large-scale opinion surveys dealing exclusively with cancer, there are a number of studies of some interest to health educators in this field.

LA POINTE *et al.* (1959), a team of psychiatrists assessing the effects of a cancer education programme in a Canadian town, describe a before-and-after study which included a questionnaire similar to those used in the Canadian national and Manchester surveys. Apart from providing confirmatory evidence for the surveys already summarized, this study offers some insight into the psychological mechanisms involved in what people "know" about cancer and into the effects of cancer education.

Additional information about the American public's knowledge of the "seven danger signals" featured in the publicity of the American Cancer Society is provided by HORN and SOLOMON (1957).

Articles by PRATT *et al.*, (1958) and SAMORA *et al.* (1962) are instructive in revealing the generally low level of health knowledge among the people studied. Equally interesting is the fact that physicians underestimated the patient's knowledge and generally failed to give a systematic explanation of prognosis, tests or treatment. Brief reference has already been made to the study by LEVINE (1962) of the psychological and social bases of anxiety about illness, but it is worthy of further comment. LEVINE found that knowledge about a disease (cancer, polio, cerebral palsy, arthritis, T. B., or birth defects) seems to be associated with fear; which is cause and which effect is by no means clear. Perhaps, he suggests, it is a vicious circle, with anxiety increasing a desire for knowledge, and the newly-acquired knowledge further increasing the anxiety. One of his major findings is that there is a positive high correlation between perceived prevalence and anxiety. It is interesting to note, however, that the age-susceptibility or prevalence factor makes little difference in the case of cancer; this disease is much feared irrespective of whether a person thinks he has a chance of getting it in the near future. The author's evidence points to the influence that similarity of social position and of personal experience has in producing similar attitudes and beliefs. In addition, the community or area in which a person lives "exerts a subtle impact on his ideas about illness", as shown by the effect that extensiveness of medical facilities has on anxiety: the more extensive they are, the less anxious a person is about getting a particular disease.

In concluding this section on attitudes to cancer, mention should be made of a survey carried out by DAVISON (1965) on a large sample of public health nurses in northern England. He found strong evidence that "many public health nurses experience feelings of frustration and despondency about cancer and that these may be passed on to laymen". Comparable studies among doctors, which would be of great importance and interest, are not yet available (but see the study by HENDERSON, WITTKOWER and LOUGHEED, 1958, referred to in Chapter 2),

References

DAVISON, R. L. (1965). Opinion of Nurses on cancer, its treatment, and its curability. *Brit. J. prev. soc. Med.* 19, 24.

HORN, D., and SOLOMON, E. S. (1957). *Perception of the seven danger signals.* Mimeo: American Cancer Society, Inc.

HORN, D., and SOLOMON, E. S. (—). *The impact of a health education program.* Mimeo: American Cancer Society, Inc.

LA POINTE, J. L., WITTKOWER, E. D., and LOUGHEED, M. N. (1959). The psychiatric evaluation of the effect of cancer education on the lay public. *Cancer* (Philad.) 12, 1200.

LEVINE, G. N. (1962). Anxiety about illness: Psychological and social bases. *J. Hlth. hum. Behav.* 3, 30.

PRATT, L., SELIGMANN, A., and READER, G. (1958). Physicians' views on the level of medical information among patients. In: *Patients, physicians and illness,* ed. by JACO E. G. (Free Press of Glencoe.) Also in *Amer. J. publ. Hlth.* 47, 1277 (1957).

SAMORA, J., SAUNDERS, L., and LARSON, R. F. (1962). Knowledge about specific diseases in four selected samples. *J. Hlth. hum. Behav.* 3, 176.

2. Studies of the Reasons for Delay in Treatment of Cancer

This chapter will be concerned not with studies specifically designed to reveal attitudes to and beliefs about cancer, but with research which has thrown a penetrating light on these matters by a less direct approach — by examining the reasons why people delay before seeking medical advice for conditions which they suspect may be caused by cancer.

Such investigations date back to the beginning of this century; but they take their present form from the study carried out by PACK and GALLO in 1938, who set the pattern by taking three months as the criterion of delay by the patient when unusual symptoms are present. For delay by the doctor, their criterion was a period of one month during which he did not refer the patient to a specialist or hospital for further examination when he was unable to make a diagnosis, or was unsuccessful in treating the condition. Most of the subsequent studies have used the same criterion of delay and have also obtained their evidence by interviewing a number of cancer patients *after* they had been referred to hospital. An important exception, however, is the study by KUTNER and GORDAN (1961). Some of the studies used methods designed to penetrate a person's awareness with more depth, a necessary stipulation, at least as a control, since it is to be expected that there are potent mechanisms at work in a person who has delayed as long as is humanly possible, using all sorts of defence mechanisms to avoid facing up to the situation. The less superficial forms of interview would seem to be especially necessary in discovering the reasons why an individual has delayed. (cf. AITKEN-SWAN and PATERSON, 1955; COBB et al., 1954; DRELLICH et al., 1956; HAMMERSCHLAG et al., 1964; HENDERSON et al., 1958; SHANDS et al., 1951; SUGAR and WATKINS, 1961; TITCHENER et al., 1956; YOUNGMAN, 1947).

The importance of these latter studies in telling us more about people's attitudes is that they represent an attempt to discover the forces motivating a person to delay or not. These forces are not solely of a practical or material nature, and to the extent that it is possible to penetrate to these presumably psychological forces, studies of this kind will increase our understanding of people's attitudes and beliefs.

A comprehensive summary of all the work done on this topic will not be given here. Instead the reader is referred to the two comprehensive reviews by KUTNER et al. (1958) and BLACKWELL (1963), summaries of which are given below with the bibliographical notes. Mention should also be made of the studies which have followed in the wake of the Pack and Gallo study at the Memorial Hospital: LEACH and ROBBINS (1947), ROBBINS et al. (1950 and 1953), also KING and LEACH (1950 and 1951). Two other series of delay studies were those carried out in conjunction with the Philadelphia Committee for the Study of Pelvic Cancer (HOWSON, 1948 a and b; 1950); HOWSON and MONTGOMERY, 1948, 1949; SCHEFFEY, 1953) and those carried out by MILLER in Michigan (MILLER, 1940, 1943, 1948; MILLER and HENDERSON, 1946, 1948). MILLER's studies are particularly interesting in that they are among the few that

take into account the doctor's evidence about delay. Delay, judged by the criteria given above, has usually been found to occur in 70%—80% of the cases where it could have been avoided.

Some of the major factors investigated in relation to delay have been: (1) the responsibility for delay; (2) psychological factors, especially fear and anxiety; (3) the individual's general level of education (4) the level of cancer education and the effect that 'knowledge' has on length of delay; (5) the site of the cancer; (6) general medical habits and their relationship to cancer; and (7) various aspects of delay by the doctor, e.g. failure to examine, pessimism, diagnostic failure, wrong treatment.

Of special importance is the finding that the mere dissemination of information will not necessarily lead to effective action; (cf. AITKEN-SWAN and PATERSON, 1955; GOLDSEN et al., 1957; HENDERSON et al., 1958; SHANDS et al., 1951; TITCHENER et al., 1956). One must also distinguish between the positive and the negative effects of fear. Fear can often be a source of motivation towards positive action that is appropriate to the situation, but it can also function in a negative way, by fostering the use of defence mechanisms (e.g. denial, repression), which only serve to put off the dreaded moment temporarily and, by non-adapted behaviour (i.e. inappropriate to the situation), make the individual even less adapted to the situation. A number of studies have suggested that this is what may happen when an individual is faced with the possibility of cancer. (cf. AITKEN-SWAN and PATERSON, 1955; BARD and SUTHERLAND, 1955; COBB et al., 1954; DRELLICH et al., 1956; KING et al., 1950; SHANDS et al., 1951; TITCHENER et al., 1956). HARMS et al., (1943) suggested that fear played only a small part, guilt being the most important factor. Unfortunately, although many studies emphasize the importance of fear in causing delay, the nature of the fear is usually left unspecified.

Of special relevance to the question of 'knowledge' and the part played by emotional factors and defence mechanisms are the studies of delay by doctors suffering from cancer (ALVAREZ 1931, BYRD 1951, ROBBINS et al. 1953). ALVAREZ's study showed considerable delay by doctors with cancer of the stomach in spite of symptoms; BYRD found that they delayed more than the general population; and ROBBINS et al. found that the doctors did not delay significantly less than the lay sample. Studies by Dublin et al. (1947, 1948 a and b) of the mortality figures for medical specialists, physicians and the general population showed that physicians died of cancer significantly less than did the general population, and surgeons significantly less than physicians. But it should be noted that these studies were concerned with death — rates and not with the temporal factor of delay.

References: Delay studies

[For studies included in the extensive reviews by KUTNER et. al. (1958) and BLACKWELL (1963) a reference only is quoted. Other studies are briefly annotated.]

AITKEN-SWAN, J., and PATERSON, R. (1955). The cancer patient: Delay in seeking advice. Brit. med. J. i, 623.

ALVAREZ, W. C. (1931). How early do physicians diagnose cancer of the stomach in themselves? J. Amer. med. Ass. 97, 77.

BARD, M., and SUTHERLAND, A. M. (1955). Psychological impact of cancer and its treatment: IV. Adaptation to radical mastectomy. Cancer, (Philad.) 8, 656.
The authors consider the "anticipatory stage", in which the person suspects that something is wrong and that it might be cancer. The influence of fear and possible delay are discussed.

BAR-MOAR, A., and DAVIES, A. M. (1960). Delay in diagnosis and treatment of cancer of the digestive tract. Harefuah, 59, 319. (Hebrew Text).
201 consecutive cases from The Rothschild Hadassah — University Hospital 1955 — 1958. Analysed according to site and responsibility for delay. 17% of the Patients delayed less than two months, 23% more than a year. The percentages for doctor — delay were 50% and 13% respectively.

BLACKWELL, B. L. (1963). The literature of delay in seeking medical care for chronic illnesses. Health Education Monographs. No 16.

Most of this review is taken up with a consideration of cancer delay, since little has been done in other fields.
It is divided into sections dealing with separate aspects of delay: existence and length of delay; site of the cancer; delay as related to personal, physical and social attributes; psychological factors associated with delay; personality of the delayer; and factors which lead to seeking care. The remainder of the work is devoted to what little has been done with respect to other chronic illnesses and psychoneuroses.

BOYCE, F. F. (1953). Certain preventable errors in the diagnosis and management of carcinoma of the stomach and the lung. Ann. Surg. 137, 864.

BRINDLEY, G. V. (1937). Carcinoma of the rectum: Factors affecting its cure. J. Amer. med. Ass. 108, 37.

BURDICK, D., and CHANATRY, F. (1954). Central New York Surgical Society Survey on Breast Carcinoma, 1920 to 1952. Cancer, (Philad.) 7, 47.

BYRD, B. F. (1951). Fatal pause in diagnosis of neoplastic disease in physician-patient. J. Amer. med. Ass. 147, 1219.

COBB, B. (1959). Emotional problems of adult cancer patients. J. Amer. Geriat. Soc. 7, 271.

COBB, B., CLARK, R. L., jr., McGUIRE, C., and HOWE, C. D. (1954). Patient — responsible delay of treatment in cancer: A social psychological study. Cancer, (Philad.) 7, 920.

COOPER, W. A. (1941). The problem of gastric cancer. *J. Amer. med. Ass.* **116**, 2125.

COOPER, W. A. (1952). Patients, physicians and gastric cancer. *J. Amer. med. Ass.* **150**, 688.

Of 687 cases (for the years 1932—1951) patients delayed for an average of eight months. There was little improvement in the decades before and after 1940. The average delay after consulting a doctor was four months. Patient-delay has its origins in ignorance, fear, and false hopes. Fundamental in this respect is the individual's reaction to illness in general.

DIDDLE, A. W. (1950). Genital cancer among women: Factors affecting its control in an urban population. *Amer. J. Obstet. Gynec.* **59**, 1373.

DRELLICH, M. G., BIEBER, I, and SUTHERLAND, A. M. (1956). The psychological impact of cancer and cancer surgery: VI. Adaptation to hysterectomy. *Cancer* **9**, 1120.

Delay is the result of fear of losing the highly-valued organ (the uterus), without which the patient feels she cannot continue in her at present adjusted and satisfying life. When the symptoms or disease are seen as a greater threat than the operation and its consequences, then she will seek treatment promptly. When operation and losing the organ are seen as a greater threat than the disease or its symptoms, she will delay.

DUBLIN, L. I., and SPIEGELMAN, M. (1947). The longevity and mortality of American physicians, 1938—1942. *J. Amer. med. Ass.* **134**, 1211.

DUBLIN, L. I., SPIEGELMAN, M., and LELAND, R. G. (1947). Longevity and mortality of physicians. *Postgrad. Med.* **2**, 188.

DUBLIN, L. I., and SPIEGELMAN, M. (1948). Mortality of medical specialists, 1938—1942. *J. Amer. med. Ass.* **137**, 1519.

FLOWERS jr., C. E., ROSS, R. A., and PRITCHETT, N. L. (1958). Delay by physician and patient in the diagnosis and treatment of pelvic cancer. *Sth. medical J.* (Bgham, Ala.) **51**, 1497.

191 cases were studied: of 131 cases of carcinoma of the cervix 70 (54%) showed no symptoms, but of the remainder 16% (21 cases) of the patients delayed, 30%

(37 cases) of the physicians delayed. For carcinoma of the endometrium the figures were 16% and 20% for patient and physician delay respectively. 75% of the cases of carcinoma of the vulva and vagina delayed. Delay in diagnosis could have been reduced in 64% of the cases by annual examination.

GOLDSEN, R. K. (1963). Patient delay in seeking cancer diagnosis: Behavioral aspects. *J. chron. Dis.* **16**, 427.

GOLDSEN, R. K., GERHARDT, P. R., and HANDY, V. H. (1957). Some factors related to patient delay in seeking diagnosis for cancer symptoms. *Cancer* (Philad) **10**, 1.

GRAY, D. B., and WARD, G. E. (1952). Delay in diagnosis of carcinoma of the stomach. *Amer. J. Surg.* **83**, 524.

GRAZIANI, E. C. (1955). Quoted in: Causes of delay in diagnosis of cancer. *J. Amer. med. Ass.* **158**, 968.

A study of one thousand patients in Peru. The figures for delay were fairly close to those in other countries. The main difference was that more responsibility for delay lay with the patient and less with the doctor. Ignorance was the most important cause of patient delay.

HAMMERSCHLAG, C. A., FISHER, S., DE COSSE, J., and KAPLAN, E. (1964). Breast symptoms and patient delay: Psychological variables involved. *Cancer* (Philad.) **17**, 1480.

Sample of forty-one patients. Tested two hypotheses: (1) that people with more sharply (subjectively) defined body boundaries would delay more, and (2) that a person who habitually employs the defence-mechanisms of denial or repression would delay more. The first hypothesis was supported, the second was not. The authors suggest that those who have a well-defined body boundary "feel more secure about their bodies, less threatened by its symptomatic alteration, and, therefore, had less need to seek immediate assistance". Furthermore, it was suggested, they delayed even more because they were less willing to enter into a submissive, dependent relationship such as exists between patient and doctor, or in a hospital.

The authors suggested that one implication of their findings is that emphasis on the personal responsibility of the individual will be most effective (if not essential) in educating such people (delayers) to seek treatment early.

HARMS, C. R., PLAUT, J. A., and OUGH-TERSON, A. W. (1943). Delay in the treatment of cancer. *J. Amer. med. Ass.* **121**, 335.

HENDERSON, J. G., WITTKOWER, E. D., and LOUGHEED, M. N. (1958). A Psychiatric investigation of the delay factor in patient to doctor presentation in cancer. *J. psychosom. Res.* **3**, 27.

One hundred cancer cases, each involving a delay of three months or more. Studied by means of a "combination of non-directive and mildly directive interview techniques". Reasons for delay were considered in relation to a large number of factors: (1) connected with the physician; (2) connected with the disease. Significant ones were — minor symptoms overlooked, previous contact with cancer (increased delay), reason for initial contact with the doctor; (3) connected with the patient, that is, attitudes to health and medical care, and personality characteristics (4) connected with cancer education. Delay is not in the main due to ignorance. The authors conclude by discussing the importance of the form that an educational campaign takes: mere presentation of facts is not sufficient. The use of fear as a basis of cancer propaganda is seriously questioned. The importance of personality and interpersonal relationships is emphasized, as also are general medical attitudes. Finally, the physicians own interpersonal relationships and attitudes are considered.

HOWSON, J. Y. (1948). Observations on the delay period in the diagnosis of pelvic cancer. *Med. Clin. N. Amer.* **32**, 1573.

HOWSON, J. Y. (1948). Pelvic cancer delay. The Organization and Observations of the Philadelphia Committee for the Study of Pelvic Cancer. *Amer. J. Obstet. Gynec.* **55**, 538.

HOWSON, J. Y. (1950). Five Procedures and Results of the Philadelphia Committee for the Study of Pelvic Cancer. *Wis. med. J.* **49**, 215.

HOWSON, J. Y., and MONTGOMERY, T. L. (1948). An attack upon the delay period in the diagnosis of pelvic cancer. *Trans. Amer. Ass. Obstet. Gynec.* **59**, 97.

HOWSON, J. Y., and MONTGOMERY, T. L. (1949). An attack upon the delay period in diagnosis of pelvic cancer. *Amer. J. Obstet. Gynec.* **57**, 1098.

KING, R. A., and LEACH, J. E. (1950). Factors contributing to delay by patients in seeking medical care. *Cancer* (Philad.) **3**, 571.

KING, R. A., and LEACH, J. E. (1951). Habits of medical care. *Cancer* (Philad.) **4**, 221.

KUTNER, B., and GORDAN, G. (1961). Seeking care for cancer. *J. Hlth hum. Behav.* **2**, 171.

KUTNER, B., MAKOVER, H. B., and OPPENHEIM, A. (1958). Delay in the diagnosis and treatment of cancer: A critical analysis of the literature. *J. chron. dis.* **7**, 95.

The authors distinguish between delay and procrastination. Delay can be unavoidable or avoidable. Only avoidable delay can be truly called procrastination; it is a failure to seek medical attention once the symptoms appear and are recognized as significant. The distinction made here is (a) between biological onset and first appearance of symptoms, and (b) between this appearance and the patient's recognition of a legitimate medical complaint.

To distinguish thus between causes of delay (insidious nature of the disease, failure to appreciate the significance of the early symptoms of cancer, and the true procrastination) is important in constructing hypotheses regarding delay and in understanding variations in behaviour within and between populations.

The authors make a very extensive review of earlier studies dealing with: (1) The prevalence of delay on the part of both patients and doctors. (2) Duration of patient-delay and doctor-delay. (3) Reasons for delay considered under several headings: patient-delay (knowledge of symptoms etc., psychological factors); physician-delay (failure to examine, diagnostic failure, wrong treatment or advice, medical attitudes and beliefs, insensitivity to the medical problem and to the patient, pessimism etc.).

The discussion points out some of the major inadequacies of the studies reviewed, and calls into question the vast majority, since they "neither provide for individual differences in the basic reasons for prompt-

ness and delay, nor for individual differences regarding the site, symptomatology,
and severity of the disease and the symptomatic onset". Finally, the authors consider
some of the problems which their review
of the literature on delay has shown to be
in need of further research.

LA COUR ANDERSEN, J., and STAKEMANN,
G. (1962). Cause of delay in diagnosis
and treatment in carcinoma of the
cervix. A study of 888 cases from
1958—1960. *Dan. med. Bull.* 9: 117.

Of the cases studied 43% were found to be
in Stage 1, 24% in stages III or IV. This
was regarded as being due to the lack of
symptoms in many cancers and to delay
by the patients. The proportion of early
cases has improved since 1942 when compared with pre- 1942, but there has been
little improvement in the past two decades.

LAWTER, D. E. DE (1948). Culpability for
delay in management of cancer. *Med.
Ann. D. C.* 17, 342. (Abstracted in *J.
Amer. med. Ass.* (1948), 138, 777,
No 1498.)

LEACH, J. E., and ROBBINS, G. F. (1947).
Delay in the diagnosis of cancer. *J.
Amer. med. Ass.* 135, 5.

MAKOVER, H. B. (1963). Patient and
physician delay in cancer diagnosis:
Medical aspects. *J. chronic Dis.* 16,
419.

Discusses several aspects of delay, many
of which are dealt with in KUTNER *et al.*
(1958), of which article Makover was a
co-author.

MILLER, N. F. (1940). Carcinoma of the
body of the uterus. *Amer. J. Obstet.
Gynec.* 40, 791.

MILLER, N. F. (1943). A consideration of
certain factors pertaining to the control of carcinoma of the cervix. *Amer.
J. Obstet. Gynec.* 46, 625.

MILLER, N. F. (1948). Carcinoma of the
uterus, ovary and tube. *J. Amer. med.
Ass.* 136, 163.

MILLER, N. F., and HENDERSON, C. W.
(1946). Corpus carcinoma. *Amer. J.
Obstet. Gynec.* 52, 894.

PACK, G. T., and GALLO, J. S. (1938). The
culpability for delay in the treatment
of cancer. *Amer. J. Cancer* 33, 443.

ROBBINS, G. F., CONTE, A. J., LEACH,

J. E., and MACDONALD, M. (1950).
Delay in diagnosis and treatment of
cancer. *J. Amer. med. Ass.* 143, 346.

ROBBINS, G. F., MACDONALD, M. C., and
PACK, G. T. (1953). Delay in the diagnosis and treatment of physicians
with cancer. *Cancer* (Philad.) 6, 624.

ROSSER, C., and KERR, J. G. (1939). Cancer of the rectum in young persons.
J. Amer. med. Ass. 113, 1192.

SCHEFFEY, L. C. (1953). The delay period
in the diagnosis of pelvic malignancy.
Obstet. and Gynec. 1, 554.

SEGSCHNEIDER, P. P., and RIEDEN, H. G.
(1960). Zur Verschleppung des Kol-
lumkarsinom. [Delay in the diagnosis
of cervical carcinoma.] *Zbl. Gynäk.*
82, 1449.

Reviews 1996 cases in years 1949—1959.
Delay in diagnosis for more than 4 weeks
was the patients' responsibility in 74.5%
of the cases, and the doctors' in 27%,
There was delay in 80.6% of the cases
(German text).

SHANDS, H. C., FINESINGER, J. E., COBB,
S., and ABRAMS, R. D. (1951). Psychological mechanisms in patients with
cancer. *Cancer* (Philad.) 4, 1159.

SIMMONS, C. C., and DALAND, E. M.
(1920). Cancer: Factors entering into
the delay in its surgical treatment.
Boston med. surg. J. 183, 298.

SIMMONS, C. C., and DALAND, E. M.
(1924). Cancer: Delay in surgical
treatment. *Boston med. surg. J.* 190,
15.

STEARNS, H. C. (1950). Discussion of
DIDDLE, A. W.: Genital cancer among
women, factors affecting its control
in an urban population. *Amer. J.
Obstet. Gynec.* 59, 1381.

STEPANOV, V. M. (1959). Causes of delayed treatment of cancer of the tongue.
Vop. Onkol 5, 216.

[Russian Text] 183 cases. 73% of patients consulted a doctor within one month,
but only 1.8% were admitted to hospital
during first month, 26.1% in first three
months, 29.7% in first five. Causes of
delay: (1) faulty diagnosis, 78%; (2) insufficient awareness of cancer among the
population 11%; (3) insidious course of
the disease 11%.

SUGAR, M., and WATKINS, C. (1961). Some
observations about patients with a

breast mass. *Cancer* (Philad.) 14, 979. A study of 50 patients prior to final diagnosis in order to discover why they delayed. Briefly stated, the conclusions were that cancer patients delayed and were depressed. Delay was not associated with knowledge of cancer symptoms nor was it caused by fear of what would be found. The non-delayer tended to show anxiety, while the delayer exhibited depression and little fear. By comparison, the patients who in fact had benign lesions were anxious and did not delay.

TAYLOR, S. G., 111, and SLAUGHTER, D. (1952). The physician and the cancer patient. *J. Amer. med. Ass.* 150, 1012. This is the sixth of a special series of articles on cancer. In it the authors discuss the improvement brought about by propaganda in bringing the patient to the doctor earlier.

TITCHENER, J. L., ZWERLING, I., GOTT-SCHALK, L., LEVINE, M., CULBERTSON, W., COHEN, S., and SILVER, H. (1956). Problem of delay in seeking surgical care. *J. Amer. med. Ass.* 160, 1187.

YOUNGMAN, N. V. (1947). Psychological aspects of the early diagnosis of cancer. *Med. J. Aust.* i, 581.

3. Having Cancer and Undergoing Treatment

This section includes a mixture of studies dealing with the emotional impact of having cancer, and various aspects of treatment, especially the psychological effects of surgery. They shed light on the meaning which cancer has for both the sick and the well.

There are attitudes and emotional reactions that spring to the fore as soon as a person suspects he has cancer, and as soon as he knows he has cancer. Information about the attitudes of cancer patients to the disease and its treatment might therefore be assumed to reflect, to some extent at least, the dormant attitudes of those who are well. And the extreme reactions to having had cancer and treatment will inevitably have repercussions upon the general public when cured patients return to circulation after leaving hospital.

Some of the most significant work on treatment and surgery for cancer has been done by SUTHERLAND and his associates, nine of whose works are listed in the bibliography. A readily-available summary of their findings and views is to be found in a chapter by SUTHERLAND in Volume 6 of *Cancer*, edited by R. W. RAVEN (1959).

An extremely thorough and interesting study of surgical patients has been made by JANIS (1958)); this work can be recommended as a reference book on the problems to be encountered in this area. For a shorter but nevertheless excellent consideration of the social and psychological implications of surgery, the reader is referred to KUTNER (1958).

Some of the factors involved in reactions to having cancer and undergoing treatment include: (1) psychological make-up of the patient; (2) habitual modes of reaction to stress, and habitual health attitudes; (3) the part of the body in which the cancer is situated and the associated guilt feelings, especially in the case of cancers of the sex organs; (4) the meaning surgery and loss of body-parts has for the individual; and (5) the various emotional reactions and defence mechanisms involved.

An important unifying concept is that distress is caused by the threat to the individual's patterns of adaptation (expectancies regarding life and significant elements of one's life, e.g. family). Where this threat cannot be dealt with, or where the idea of cancer cannot be integrated into one's patterns of adaptation, the situation can only be dealt with by a defence mechanism, whether it be attack or retreat.

The importance of the body-part affected by cancer lies in the meaning and

significance it has for the person concerned. This is what has been referred to
as "body-image". Thus the same type of
cancer and treatment can affect different
people in different ways. Perhaps the
most obvious example in this field is the
female breast. The possibility of surgical
removal is not merely the prospect of a
physical trauma, but also an assault on
the woman's own image of her femininity.
SUTHERLAND's work, for example, has
shown that reaction against surgical removal of the breast was most extreme in
those women for whom their femininity
played a large part in their relations with
society.

References: Having cancer and cancer treatment

ABRAMS, R. D., and FINESINGER, J. E.
(1953). Guilt reactions in patients with
cancer. *Cancer* (Philad.) **6**, 474.

Sample of 60 unselected cancer patients.
Attitudes of patients and doctors were
studied by interviewing. Patients need to
find a cause for their illness: 93% of the
patients showed feelings of guilt, due
mainly to cancer being looked upon as
unclean. Medical staff, too, showed special
attitudes concerning cancer. Guilt feelings
were responsible for (1) delay, (2) emotionally negative attitudes or feelings, and
(3) patients' inability to communicate. The
authors conclude by considering measures
taken to relieve the feelings of guilt.

ADSETT, C. A. (1963). Emotional reactions
to disfigurement from cancer therapy.
Canad. med. Ass. J. **89**, 385.

This article summarizes conclusions from
studies contained in this section of the
present bibliography.

AITKEN-SWAN, J., and EASSON, E. C.
(1959). Reactions of cancer patients on
being told their diagnosis. *Brit. med. J.*
i, 779.

231 selected cancer patients were told their
diagnosis. Between a week to a month later
their reactions to being told were checked:
66% were glad to know the truth, 7%
disapproved, and 19% denied they had
ever been told. None of the 35 family
doctors who were asked reported any
undesirable effect caused by the patients
having learned the diagnosis.

BARD, M. (1952). The sequence of emotional reactions in radical mastectomy
patients. *Publ. Hlth. Rep.* (Wash.) **67**,
1144. See BARD and SUTHERLAND
(1955) below, and SUTHERLAND (1959).

BARD, M., and SUTHERLAND, A. M. (1955).
Psychological impact of cancer and its
treatment: IV Adaptation to radical
mastectomy. *Cancer* (Philad.) **8**, 656.
See SUTHERLAND (1959). Of special interest in this study is the consideration of the
significance of the breasts and their relation to the individual woman's femininity.
No generalizations can be made about the
response of an individual to cancer of the
breast and mastectomy; each case must be
considered in the light of the individual's
adjustment to the important areas of life
(death, sex, family etc.) and the values she
has concerning them.

BELLAK, L. (Ed.) (1952). *Psychology of
physical illness: Psychiatry applied to
medicine, surgery and the specialities.*
London: J. & A. Churchill Ltd., New
York: Grune & Stratton Inc. (Chapters
of particular interest are annotated
under entries for Meerloo and Rosen).

BRANT, C. S., VOLK, H., and KUTNER, B.
(1958). Psychological preparation for
surgery. *Publ. Hlth. Rep.* (Wash.) **73**,
1001.

A study of 50 patients. There is a need
to deal with the anxieties surrounding the
pre- and post-operative periods. Recommendations are made.

COBB, B. (1959). Emotional problems of
adult cancer patients. *J. Amer. Geriat.
Soc.* **7**, 274.

40 patients. 3 major categories of
stress: (1) the meaning of cancer for the
individual; (2) the change from active to
passive life; (3) separation, temporary or
permanent. The doctor-patient relationship is considered in the light of these
stresses.

DRELLICH, M. G., BIEBER, I., and SUTHER-
LAND, A. M. (1956). The psychological
impact of cancer and cancer surgery:
VI Adaptation to hysterectomy. *Cancer* (Philad.) **9**, 1120.

See SUTHERLAND (1959). This article is of special interest for consideration of the psychological significance of the uterus.

DYK, R. B., and SUTHERLAND, A. M. (1956). Adaptation of the spouse and other family members to the colostomy patient. *Cancer* (Philad.) 9, 123. See SUTHERLAND (1959).

GERLE, B., LUNDEN, G., and SANDBLOM, P. (1960). The patient with inoperable cancer from the psychiatric and social standpoints. *Cancer* (Philad.) 13, 1206.
101 cases. Deals with the question of telling the patient his diagnosis. Found that fear of death does not seem to be the main cause of worry, but rather the pain associated with cancer.

GREENE jr., W. A., YOUNG, L. E., and SWISHER, S. N. (1956). Psychological factors and reticuloendothelial disease: II Observations on a group of women with lymphomas and leukemias. *Psychosom. Med.* 18, 284.
The authors found that the predominant emotional reaction was shame and not guilt. They suggest that this may be a characteristic response to this type of cancer as opposed to neoplasms.

JANIS, I. L. (1958). *Psychological Stress: Psychoanalytic and behavioral studies of surgical patients.* New York: John Wiley & Sons Inc.
Evidence from three sources: intensive case-studies of thirty patients, a second study by means of questionnaires of several hundred recent surgical cases, and the psychoanalysis of a patient who underwent surgery. The work aims firstly to bring out the *theoretical* implications of the surgical situation by an examination of the way people respond to stressful events in their lives. The second aim is to emphasise the *practical* implications, especially those concerned with (a) medical management, which must take into account the needs of the patients, (b) the better prediction of how a patient will tolerate stress, and (c) effective psychological preparation for surgery.
One of the main findings was that someone faced with the threat of mutilation or death will revert (regress) to the emotional responses employed and found satisfactory in stress situations of early childhood. The other major finding was

that post-operative reactions will depend on pre-operative anxiety. The most extreme emotional disturbance will appear post-operatively where the patient has had very high or very low anticipatory (pre-operative) fear. Those who exhibit a moderate (medium) degree of pre-operative fear exhibit least post-operative disturbance.

KLINE, N. S., and SOBIN, J. (1951). The psychological management of cancer cases. *J. Amer. med. Ass.* 146, 1547.
The author considers whether a patient should be told the diagnosis, and types of reaction to knowing that he has cancer — flight from the disease, over-reaction to, and obsessive preoccupation with the disease.

KUTNER, B. (1958). Surgeons and their patients: A study in social perception. In, *Patients, Physicians and Illness*, ed. by E. G. JACO. Glencoe (Ill.): Free Press.
In the course of an excellent article the author deals with (1) the interpersonal relationships in surgery; (2) some social and psychological needs of surgeons: the operator's role; and (3) the social and psychological needs of patients: the meaning of surgery, social traumata of operations, the search for meaning, psychological preparation, the perception of the surgeon's role, and the implications for medical education and research.

MEERLOO, J. A. M. (1954). Psychological implications of malignant growth: A survey of hypotheses. *Brit. J. med. Psychol.* 27, 210.
Hypotheses put forward by the author deal with: psychosomatic aspects of the disease, fear of cancer created by propaganda, the psychological impact of surgical lesions, and the psychological problems of the investigator. Also considered are the psychological mechanisms of fear, frustration and denial at work in the doctor and patient when confronted with the possibility of cancer.

MEERLOO, J. A. M., and ZECKEL, A. (1952). Psychiatric problems of malignancy. In: *Psychology of physical illness: Psychiatry applied to medicine, surgery, and the specialities*, ed. by L. BELLAK. London: J. & A. Churchill Ltd.; New York: Grune & Stratton Inc.

This short but useful chapter deals with the patient's attitudes concerning malignancies and the emotional significance they and the site of the malignancy have for him. The importance of the attitudes of the doctor and of the patient's family is also discussed.

MENZER, D., MORRIS, T., GATES, P., SABBATH, J., ROBEY, H., PLAUT, T., and STURGIS, S. H. (1957). Patterns of emotional recovery from hysterectomy. *Psychosom. Med.* 19, 379.

26 patients studied. Found that a crucial factor associated with post-operative reaction was the habitual way the patient handled fear and other dificult life situations prior to operation. Also of importance was the patient's attitude to femininity.

MEYER, B. C. (1958). Some psychiatric aspects of surgical practice. *Psychosom. Med.* 20, 203.

Considers the psychological characteristics of the patient and situation prior to surgery; pre-surgery psychological manifestations; the post-operative period; psychological and therapeutic aspects of mutilation; the patient-surgeon relationship.

ORBACH, C. E., and SUTHERLAND, A. M. (1954). Acute depressive reactions to surgical treatment for cancer. In: *Depression*, ed. by P. H. HOCH and J. ZUBIN. New York: Grune & Stratton. See SUTHERLAND (1959).

RENNEKER, R., and CUTLER, M. (1952). Psychological problems of adjustment to cancer of the breast. *J. Amer. med. Ass.* 148, 833.

The dual psychological conflict confronting a woman with breast cancer arises from the need for adjustment to breast mutilation, and the need for adjustment to invasion of her body by a potentially deadly disease. The emotional meaning that the breasts have for a woman is important.

ROSEN, V. H. (1952). Psychiatric problems in general surgery. In: *Psychology of physical illness: Psychiatry applied to medicine, surgery and the specialities,* ed. by L. BELLAK. London: J. & A. Churchill Ltd.

An excellent chapter dealing with the threat of danger involved in surgery, the emo-

tional responses to danger, the process of undergoing surgery, and various specific aspects of surgery, such as chest surgery and amputation of a limb.

ROSS, W. S. (1965). *The climate is hope — How they triumphed over cancer.* New York: Prentice-Hall, Inc.

Not a research work, but throws interesting light on the attitudes to cancer of those treating it — and suffering from it. (See further entry in Chapter 12).

SHANDS, H. C., FINESINGER, J. E., COBB, S., and ABRAMS, R. D. (1951). Psychological mechanisms in patients with cancer. *Cancer* (Philad.) 4, 1159.

An important article dealing in some depth with the integration by the individual of the distressing information that he has cancer. The processes and levels by which this is achieved, the part played by defence-mechanisms and by pain are discussed, as is the doctor-patient relationship. Adaptation to the new situation will result in the reduction of anxiety; adaptation should be aimed at, even though much distress may be involved in the process.

SUTHERLAND, A. (1952). Psychological impact of cancer surgery. *Publ. Hlth. Rep.* (Wash.) 67, 1139. See SUTHERLAND (1959).

SUTHERLAND, A. (1956). Psychological impact of cancer and its therapy. *Med. Clin. N. Amer.* 40, 705. See SUTHERLAND (1959).

SUTHERLAND, A. M. (1959). Psychological impact of cancer and its therapy. In: *Cancer,* vol. 6, ed. by R. W. RAVEN. London: Butterworth & Co., (Publ.) Ltd.

In this article SUTHERLAND summarizes many of the general findings of his own and his co-workers' studies. The experience of having cancer is a special and severe form of stress involving the threat of death, or of mutilation, or of both. Many fundamental, underlying, emotionally-charged convictions are brought to the surface in a cancer patient. The experience of having cancer cannot be separated from the experience of its therapy, and each type of operation has its own special problems (see the separate articles in this bibliography). The ill-effects of the stress caused by threat of death or mutilation consequent on surgery are produced mainly in four ways: (1) by disrupting or threatening to disrupt a major pattern of adaptation to life; certain organs (e.g. sexual) often play an important part here; (2) by activating a system of beliefs, assumptions, values and other notions which become explicit determinants of action (e.g. concerning the function of a particular organ); (3) by attacking an organ whose function has been guiltily maintained throughout the patient's life; and (4) by constituting one more serious difficulty in the life of a person already overloaded with frustration and sorrow. All the individual's behaviour is geared to minimizing the disruption of established patterns of adaptation to life as he sees it. These patterns include activity, beliefs, values, orientations etc.; physical organs play a greater or lesser part in this adaptation, and so

threat involving these organs will result in the use of mechanisms of defence proportional to the perceived disruption and possible loss. This view of the behaviour of the patient is considered in the various conditions of the pre-operative, surgical, reparative and post-operative phases.

SUTHERLAND, A. M., and ORBACH, C. E. (1953). Psychological impact of cancer and cancer surgery: 11 Depressive reactions associated with surgery for cancer. *Cancer (Philad.)* 6, 958. See SUTHERLAND (1959).

SUTHERLAND, A. M., ORBACH, C. E., DYK, R. B., and BARD, M. (1952). The psychological impact of cancer and cancer surgery: 1 Adaptation to the dry colostomy; preliminary report and summary of findings. *Cancer* (Philad.) 5, 857. See SUTHERLAND (1959).

4. Delay in Seeking Treatment for Diseases other than Cancer

This chapter will consider the evidence regarding delay in treatment for other serious diseases, since it is important to know whether or not delay in seeking care for cancer is merely a reflection of general patterns of behaviour and particularly medical habits, or whether cancer delay is a special case in which unreasonable attitudes result in abnormally long delay.

Evidence that delay or non-delay in seeking care for cancer is determined by a person's general pattern of behaviour concerning medical matters receives support from several studies (COBB *et al.*, 1954; GOLDSEN *et al.*, 1957; HENDERSON *et al.*, 1958; and KING and LEACH, 1950). Contrary evidence comes from SUGAR and WATKINS (1961) and TITCHENER *et al.*, (1956), who found that non-cancer cases delayed less than cancer cases, but did not analyse their findings in terms of general health habits. The importance of such an analysis is brought out by GOLDSEN (1963), who further analysed the findings of KUTNER and GORDAN (1961) that people with cancer symptoms delayed more than those with non-cancer

symptoms. GOLDSEN showed that those who did not delay when they had symptoms suggestive of cancer had "good medical habits", and of those who delayed, significantly fewer fell into this category. This question needs more study to distinguish between delay in cancer and non-cancer cases, and also between those with good and bad medical habits.

Studies of delay in the treatment of other diseases are almost non-existent. BLACKWELL (1963) found a few tangentially relevant works concerned with cardiac cases.

The most relevant of these was by JÄRVINEN (1960), who found that delay was much greater in the case of males following an attack of acute myocardial infarction, and was also greater when the attack occurred at home.

WITTKOWER (1949) found that delay in the treatment of tuberculosis resulted from the unwillingness of the patient to admit that he was ill, and from his denial of the seriousness of his condition. BAUMERT and HOPPE (1958) found the same. (cf. similar reasons for not taking part in

a tuberculosis X-ray programme (HOCH-
BAUM, 1959) and a poliomyelitis vaccination programme (ROSENSTOCK *et al.*,
1959).

References: Delay in diseases other than cancer

BAUMERT, G., and HOPPE, R. (1958). Un-
tersuchungen über den Einfluß sozialer
Faktoren in der Tuberkulose-Therapie.
[Investigations of the influence of social factors on the treatment of tuber-
culosis]. *Köln. Z. Soziol. Soz.-Psychol.*,
Suppl. 3, 219. *(Recorded in sociological
abstracts*, 1959, 7, No. 6712).

COBB, B., CLARK, R. L., McGUIRE, C.,
and HOWE, C. D. (1954).

GOLDSEN, R. K. (1963).

GOLDSEN, R. K., GERHARDT, P. R., and
HANDY, V. H. (1957).

HENDERSON, J. G., WITTKOWER, E. D.,
and LOUGHEED, M. N. (1958).

HOCHBAUM, G. M. (1959). What they
believe and how they behave. *Int. J.
Hlth. Educ.* 2, 43.

JÄRVINEN, K. A. J. (1960). Physical activity of patients after the onset of
acute cardiac infarction. *Brit. med. J.*
i, 922.

KING, R. A., and LEACH, J. E. (1950).

KUTNER, B., and GORDAN, G. (1961).

ROSENSTOCK, I. M., DERRYBERRY, M., and
CARRIGER, B. K. (1959). Why people
fail to seek poliomyelitis vaccination.
Publ. Hlth. Rep. (Wash.) 74, 98,

SUGAR, M., and WATKINS, C. (1961).

TITCHENER, J. L., ZWERLING, I., GOTT-
SCHALK, L., LEVINE, M., CULBERTSON,
W., COHEN, S., and SILVER, H. (1956).

WITTKOWER, E. D. (1949). *A psychiatrist
looks at tuberculosis*. London: The
National Association for the Prevention of Tuberculosis.

More details of the papers for which only
the authors are quoted above are given in
the list of references at the end of Chapter 2.

5. The Individual in Society and Being Ill

This chapter looks at studies of what
is understood by "being ill", since this is
an integral part of the situation that the
health educator must have before him in
designing and executing his programme.
What is it that society accepts as illness?
What does it mean to the healthy person
and the sick? How does hospitalization
affect the patient and his immediate circle,
and what part does the doctor play in this
complex interaction of factors?

PARSONS' theoretical approach has stim-
ulated a great deal of work on the meaning of illness and its consequences. In his
book, *The Social System* (1952), he tries
to explain the particular social system
which operates when a person is ill. The
normal member of society has certain
obligations to society and *vice versa;*
when he becomes ill, society releases him
from some of his obligations and imposes

others on him. One of the new obligations involved in being ill (or, in the current jargon, as a result of assuming the
sick-role) is that of getting well again.
Hence the importance of the part played
by the doctor in this special social system.
PARSONS and subsequent authors (e.g.
MECHANIC, 1962; BRUHN, 1962; HOL-
LINGSHEAD and REDLICH, 1958; SUCH-
MAN, 1965) have developed various aspects of the theory of roles (see also
Chapter 9), an important element in our
understanding of how individuals and
groups interact in the face of disease.

There have been several studies of the
meaning of health and illness for people
living in various family and socioeconomic conditions. Sociological and anthropological studies emphasize the social
nature of the sick-role, and the ways in
which communities employ myths to fill

the gaps in their medical knowledge. This is particularly relevant to our understanding of the origin and persistence of prejudices and assumptions that are not based on objective reality.

The concept of the sick-role is of particular importance to health educators. It refers not only to the partially-isolated individual (e. g. as a patient in hospital) but also to the study of all that illness means for society, and for the individual as a member of that society. It seeks to define the breakdowns in proper functioning, either physical or mental, which are accepted as illness and so permit the individual to assume the sick-role. It also tries to clarify the position which illness occupies in the larger hierarchy of role-demands. What society expects of the sick person varies considerably from country to country and even from region to region in the same country. In one place, he is expected to stop work and seek treatment as soon as certain accepted symptoms appear; in another, with a tradition of stoicism, he is expected to work on and fulfil his normal tasks until he is physically incapable of carrying on. The health educator who, in such a community, seeks to introduce prompt referral to a doctor for symptoms which are in no way disabling faces an impossible task unless he is aware of the accepted norms of behaviour in the community and bases his efforts on gradual change. Those who prematurely introduce screening of healthy people for pre-cancerous lesions in such communities must be prepared to face a blank wall of incomprehension; for they cannot expect their own values to be accepted when they run counter to the whole structure of roles in the recipient society.

The attitudes of the medical profession are of paramount importance in any health education programme. Not only is active co-operation by the profession a vital element of such work, but the attitudes of doctors and educators to the problem must also be in agreement if the programme is to have any hope of success. Doctors play an important part in the social definition of the sick-role, and in the general education of the public on matters of health. The close personal relationship of doctors with their patients makes them a potent source of influence on the general public. (See chapter 11, section on "The Communicator"). That influence can be for good or ill, according to the doctors' own attitudes to the problems at hand and to the solution envisaged by the educator. Unless the doctors in the community can be persuaded to lend their support, whether moral or practical, to a public education programme, it cannot succeed.

Reviews of Sociological aspects of disease and medicine.

In other sections of this bibliography, we have found it necessary to list references to important studies at some length. Fortunately, however, in this important section dealing with the psychological and social implications of illness and medical care, it is possible to list a few excellent works which either review particular areas of the field, or cover a considerable part of the whole field in a collection of invited or reprinted chapters by well-known workers.

Two excellent recent reviews of work in sociology and anthropology in relation to medicine have been written by POLGAR (1962) and SCOTCH (1965); the latter covers the two years succeeding Polgar's review. An earlier review was done by CAUDILL (1953).

Five books which are highly recommended to the reader are *Health, Culture, and Community*, edited by B. D. PAUL (1955), *Patients, Physicians and Illness*, edited by E. G. JACO (1958), *Sociological Studies of Health and Sickness*, edited by

D. APPLE (1960), and *Handbook of Me-dical Sociology*, edited by H. E. FREE-MAN *et al.*, (1963). Together these four works provide one hundred and thirteen chapters or articles. A book which takes a different form is *Sociology in Medicine* by M. W. SUSSER and W. WATSON (1962). Unlike the others, this is not a collection of readings, but a well-documented con-sideration of the interaction of sociology and medicine in both peasant and in-dustrialized societies. STOECKLE, ZOLA and DAVIDSON (1963) have made a useful

review of studies relevant to the decision of patients to visit the doctor.

Finally, there are two bibliographies which merit special mention. The first is by MARION PEARSALL (1963), and the se-cond, included as a chapter in FREEMAN *et al.* (1963) was compiled by O. SIM-MONS. They provide an excellent starting point for anyone who wishes to undertake library research into any aspect of the literature concerned with the social set-ting of disease.

References: The individual in society and being ill

APPLE, D. (Ed.) (1960). *Sociological stud-ies of health and sickness*. New York: McGraw-Hill Book Co.

BRUHN, J. (1962). An operational ap-proach to the sick-role concept. *Brit. J. med. Psychol.* 35, 289.

CAUDILL, W. (1953). Applied anthropol-ogy in medicine. Chapter in anthro-pology today: an encyclopedic inven-tory, ed. by A. L. KROEGER. Chicago: University Illinois Press.

FREEMAN, H. E., LEVINE, S., and REEDER, L. G. (Eds.) (1963). *Handbook of medical sociology*. New Jersey: Pren-tice-Hall.

HOLLINGSHEAD, A. B., and REDLICH, F. C. (1958). *Social class and mental illness*. New York: John Wiley & Sons.

JACO, E. G. (Ed.) (1958). *Patients, phy-sicians and illness: Sourcebook in be-havioral science and medicine*. Glen-coe (Ill.): The Free Press.

MECHANIC, D. (1962). The concept of illness behavior. *J. chron. Dis.* 15, 189.

PARSONS, T. (1952) *The social system*. London: Tavistock Publications. (See also chapter in JACO 1958).

PAUL, B. D. (Ed.) (1955). *Health, culture, and community*. New York: Russell Sage Foundation.

PEARSALL, MARION. (1963). *Medical be-havioral science: A Selected biblio-graphy of cultural anthropology, so-cial psychology, and sociology in me-dicine*. Lexington, Kentucky: Univer-sity Kentucky Press.

POLGAR, S. (1962). Health and human behavior: Areas of interest common to the social and medical sciences. *Curr. Anthropol.* 3, 159.

SCOTCH, N. A. (1963). Medical anthro-pology. In: *Biennial review of anthro-pology*, ed. by B. J. SIEGEL. Stanford, California: Stanford University Press.

STOECKLE, J. D., ZOLA, I. K., and DAVID-SON, G. E. (1963). On going to see the doctor, The contributions of the patient to the decision to seek medical aid. *J. chron. Dis.* 16, 975.

SUSSER, M. W., and WATSON, W. (1962). *Sociology in medicine*. London: Ox-ford University Press.

The Behaviour of the Individual and Motivation

This section of the monograph is treated differently from the rest. It has been possible in other sections to prepare either detailed bibliographies of published work on the study of attitudes to cancer, as in chapter 1, which called for no more than an accurate presentation of what facts have so far been uncovered; or to present a guide to some of the accessible and up-to-date reviews of research in other disciplines, as in Chapter 5, in which our aim has been to refer readers to authoritative compendia of information rather than to provide a substantial commentary of our own.

In the present section, however, dealing with the psychological and socio-psychological aspects of what the health educator and physician must regard as inappropriate behaviour, we have found it impossible either to present a guide to reliable reviews of the situation, or to attempt the task of summarizing all current trends of thinking. There is so much disagreement among specialists within the field of psychology that the nonspecialist would be courting disaster by advocating one line of argument or another.

In this chapter, therefore, we have not tried to give a balanced view of psychological theory, but to present a number of pointers to the explanations offered for certain types of behaviour. Given the format of this monograph, such a review cannot hope to be comprehensive, but we hope it will be stimulating to someone coming new into the field of cancer education and provocative to those who have been involved in it for some time. It is *not* intended for the specialist.

The emphasis throughout is on pointing the way to published work which seeks to explain the barriers to rational action. We know that there are people who, when faced with disturbing signs or symptoms, visit the doctor promptly as a means of resolving their anxieties. But people of this kind are *not* the ones who pose real problems for the health educator. Our concern is necessarily with the people who do not behave in the most sensible way when threatened by the signs and symptoms of disease.

Whenever a health-educator plans a campaign or a lesson, he does so with certain preconceived notions about man's nature and mode of functioning. When he makes appeals of an emotional, rational or other kind, he is, in fact, presuming that man is of such a nature that he will respond to the appeals in a particular manner. The health-educator does not sit down to have a philosophical or psychological "think" about the nature of man as a preliminary to his work, though his campaign might sometimes benefit if he did so. MENDELSOHN (1964) does precisely this from the point of view of those involved in the planning and directing of public education in safety campaigns; his controversial but stimulating remarks could be read with equal profit by those involved in public education about cancer.

One of the most important reservations to keep in mind in considering any psychological treatise is that the author is dealing with an extremely complex being in an equally complex situation. In consequence, whatever starting point he takes, whatever aspect he considers, whatever concept he uses, and whatever tools or methods of study he employs, he is limited to a greater or lesser degree in the overall coverage of his subject and in the generality of his conclusions. This should, however, not prevent him from always attempting to see man, his behaviour, and his environment as an interacting whole.

Man is a complex of inherited physical and psychical characteristics and dispositions, able to learn new pieces of behaviour and concepts, and greatly influenced by his social environment. Such a description of man includes those aspects usually considered by psychologists under the headings of heredity, drives, personality, learning, motivation, perception, cognition, and the social and behavioural concepts of groups, roles, communication, and attitudes. It is with these that we will be dealing in the succeeding chapters.

Reference

MENDELSOHN, H. A. (1964). A critical review of the literature and a proposed theory. In: *The Denver symposium on mass communications research for safety*, ed by. M. BLUMENTHAL.: National Safety Council, U.S.A.

6. Motivation

Probably one of the most obscure and at the same time most important concepts in psychology is that of motivation. It is obscure to the extent that it is ill-defined, and important in so far as it asks the key question of psychology: why does man behave as he does? The definitions of motivation are as diverse as the approaches to this question, and as the differences in emphasis placed on various aspects of behaviour. Psychologists have, however, been interested to a greater or lesser degree in motivation of behaviour as demonstrated by new or increased activity, and/or they have been concerned with the reasons or causes (i.e. the "why") of behaviour.

The structure of those theories concerned with the "why" of behaviour depends to a large extent on the sample of behaviour that is examined. Thus "drive" theories of motivation, that see all behaviour as the effect (direct, or indirect e.g. as a result of learning) of a number of primitive drives (hunger, thirst, sex, etc.), are proposed mainly by those psychologists concerned with lower animals.

On the other hand, those psychologists who are especially interested in man in his social setting will see his behaviour as influenced by his surroundings in the form, for example, of social roles, reference groups etc.

One of the most pervasive ideas about motivation is that it can be compared to a hydraulic system: pressure or level builds up until it flows over in the form of behaviour. Such a view was taken by early psycho-analysts and appears to be generally supported by many theorists and by everyday experience. This, surely, is something of an oversimplification; the inadequacy of the hydraulic analogy would appear to lie in its failure to take into account (1) the effect of learning on the establishment of the hydraulic set-up (often called "equilibration" or "equilibrium"), and (2) the influence of factors external to the person, especially, in the case of man, social influences.

For the present purpose, however, it has been decided to discuss a few important aspects of motivation, rather than to concentrate on theoretical issues.

(i) Conflict

A frequent characteristic of behaviour is conflict, which can be either between possible but incompatible actions, or between ways of doing them (see COFER and APPLEY, 1964). Some people are able to resolve conflict by appropriate action, but it is with those in whom conflict is not so resolved that cancer education is most concerned.

Two of the most prominent researchers into conflict have been LEWIN (1931, 1935, 1938; also LEEPER, 1943) and MILLER (1944, 1951; DOLLARD and MILLER, 1950). LEWIN analysed conflict in terms of overlapping fields, forces and directed movements in the psychological space that included the person concerned and all he, the individual, considered to be important to himself. This view led to a classification of conflict into three main types: —

1. *approach — approach:* i. e. the positive attraction of two incompatible goals.

2. *avoidance — avoidance:* i. e. both choices are unattractive.

3. *approach — avoidance:* i. e. the ambivalent situation in which a person is both attracted and repelled by the same object.

These three types of conflict have different characteristics. In the *approach—approach* situation, the conflict is only really a problem to the extent that the attraction to the two goals or objects is nearly equal, since otherwise the more attractive one would soon predominate over the less attractive. The most important characteristic of *avoidance—avoidance* is that the person in such a situation will attempt to flee from both objects, and can only be kept from doing so by means of barriers (physical or psychological). Another characteristic of such conflict is that, unlike *approach—avoidance* and to some extent *approach—approach*, the conflict is never resolved and is often increased. There is often vacilla-tion between the two undesirable goals. Having said that the conflict is never resolved, two reservations are necessary: (1) that the barriers must remain impenetrable, and (2) the individual may escape psychologically from the situation. An example of such psychological escape is the use of defence-mechanisms by a person who experiences great fear or anxiety whichever way he turns (e.g. a woman's going to see a doctor versus living with the possibility that she has cancer — she may deny that she has any symptoms, or rationalize them away, etc.). A typical reaction of both animals and men in grossly fearful and inescapable situations is to "freeze" and do nothing.

The approach—avoidance experience is perhaps the most common of all; very rarely does an action seem attractive from all points of view. No barrier is involved here, since one is attracted towards the goal, but also kept from it by the repelling force associated with the goal. Even more so than in *avoidance—avoidance*, vacillation is the characteristic of this conflict. Such conflict is particularly interesting in the light of Miller's work in analysing conflict in terms of gradients of approach and avoidance. He has postulated and demonstrated a number of important hypotheses:

(1) the tendencies to approach or to avoid increase the nearer the person is to the goal; hence more effort is made at the end of a course to obtain a desired goal; but, on the other hand, one backs away more from an undesirable or noxious goal the closer one gets to it. (2) The tendency to back away increases much more than does the tendency to approach, the nearer to the goal one is. A consequence of this is that to reduce the tendency to avoidance (e.g. by removing a frightening warning-signal) will result in a greater lessening of tension than will be obtained by increasing the degree of

attraction to the goal. (3) The strengths of the approach and avoidance tendencies depend on the underlying drives, and so can be varied. Because of the characteristics of the two gradients, changes in either of them will have different results, as mentioned already in (2) (see LEWIN, 1958). A small but important point is that the distance from a goal is not strictly or solely spatial, but psychological or temporal. Important in any situation where there are both positive and negative motivations is the level of achievement to which a person aspires.

Mention has already been made of the vacillation or hesitation that may occur, especially where there is conflict between two attractive goals, or between the attractive and non-attractive aspects of the same goal. This is a sufficiently common phenomenon to merit special mention. In this situation there is a critical point at which the attractive and repulsive qualities of an action will seem equal to the individual. At such a point he will hesitate most, perhaps even stopping altogether. This is the moment of greatest indecision, and thus most crucial in any decision to go on or go back. To continue pursuing a course of action after this point of commitment can result in increased suffering, pain, loss, cost, or whatever is discouraging him from going towards the goal. An example of this would be the build-up of hesitation when someone finds that he has a symptom suggestive of a feared disease. He will hesitate and put off going to the doctor, and when he finally does reach the consulting-room he experiences a mounting conflict between, on the one hand, telling the doctor, with all the possible sequelae of telling (e.g. being told he has cancer, hospitalization, painful treatment, or even death), and, on the other hand, saying nothing and being spared (for the moment!) all such unpleasant results.

There are, of course, those who cope with the situation and find appropriate relief from these conflicts by putting themselves into the hands of doctors whom they trust. Fortunately, there are many such people, but the numbers who do not are still distressingly large, and it is with the psychological background to their inaction that we have been concerned here.

(ii) Frustration and reactions to frustration

In considering conflict we have, in fact, been dealing with those situations where one or other possibility open to a person is hindered or frustrated. A great amount of work has been done in studying the effects of frustration in animals and, to a lesser extent, in man.

One of the earliest examples was observed in PAVLOV's laboratories (PAVLOV, 1927): a dog was fed after being shown a circle but not after an ellipse; as the difference between them became less, the animal found it increasingly difficult to discriminate between them, until finally its behaviour deteriorated to such a degree that the effects have been called "experimental neurosis". Without examining in detail the pros or cons of such a description, we can note the interesting effects of ambiguous stimuli which are sometimes associated with reward and sometimes with punishment, and ask whether there are not some similarities with possible symptoms of feared diseases. For a fuller treatment of "experimental neurosis" see WATERS *et al.*, (1960). At the human level, psychoanalysts have attempted to show that neuroses in adult life stem primarily from unresolved conflicts in childhood. There is evidence that conflicts are at the root of psychosomatic ailments.

Although the suspicion of cancer does not necessarily produce the extreme forms of reaction to frustration discussed here, these possible reactions are discussed in some detail to provide a theoretical background to the problems of those who behave unrealistically when confronted with the threat of cancer. Different research workers have emphasized different reactions to frustration, some of which are considered below:

(a) Repression. This can most easily be described as "motivated forgetting". The extreme case of this is amnesia which occurs when a motive is too threatening and so results in high anxiety. There is evidence for this in the Yale communication studies (e.g. HOVLAND *et al.*, 1953. See (i) p. 46 of present work) and in studies of perception (see chapter 7), as well as in the classical psychoanalytical writings (see FREUD, 1937). A relevant example is the denial by a cured patient that she has ever had cancer or been told the diagnosis (AITKEN-SWAN and EASSON, 1959).

(b) Rationalization. Another way of dealing with a threatening situation is by explaining away the fear-provoking behaviour. This is called "rationalization", for which abundant evidence exists in everyday life; for example, the woman who finds "good" reasons for not going to see her doctor, or who finds alternative but less frightening explanations for a possible cancer symptom.

(c) Projection. This, basically, is the placing of responsibility for one's own unwanted motives (which may be repressed) or behaviour on others. Such a defence is often to be found in prejudiced people who put the blame for their own views on the group they are prejudiced against. An example of this would be a woman who claims that she derived her attitudes opposed to cytological examination for cancer from her doctor.

(d) Aggression. Probably one of the most common reactions to frustration is aggression. Such a reaction is not strictly a defence mechanism in that it need not be covert, but it is designed to defend the person frustrated, and it may lead to unconscious reactions. For example, the aggression may be turned towards oneself in self-blame, or it may be displaced and directed against something else. Aggression is a frequent component in the reactions of a patient who has undergone major surgery.

(e) Displacement. By this mechanism a person is able to vent his (hostile) feelings on someone other than the frustrating person. This is the basis of the "scapegoat" system. An obvious example of displacement in the field of medical care is the anger which is sometimes visited on doctors when they are unable to help a patient who has delayed too long in seeking help.

(f) Reaction formation. As the name implies, this defence involves reacting to the fear-arousing situation by overtly going to the opposite extreme in one's behaviour or expressed feelings (while the real ones are repressed). It has been suggested that the good response by people to appeals by cancer organisations for support and for voluntary help might be a case of reaction formation.

(g) Regression. This is *par excellence* a psychoanalytical concept (FREUD, 1949) and refers to the phenomenon of a person who, when faced with a problem, employs methods which were formerly successful but which are no longer suitable. Regression may be seen in a person's way of dealing with his environment when under great stress. For example, before or after undergoing a major surgical operation, a patient may adopt the purely passive role of childhood in relation to his doctors and treatment (see SUTHERLAND, 1959).

(h) Fixation. The final defence-mechanism to concern us here is the response, or lack of it, to a situation in which the individual moves neither forward nor back; he appears to "freeze". This is also a psychoanalytical concept, but much animal-laboratory evidence is available (e.g. MAIER, 1949, 1956) to show the fixating effect of frustration. An example of this type of defence-mechanism would be a man who for a long period of time, and in spite of contra-indications, had recourse to quack-medicines for cancer symptoms.

(iii) Fear or anxiety

One of the most potent barriers against escaping from a frustrating situation, and one of the most frequent stimuli leading to avoidance, is fear. MOWRER (1960 a and b) has put fear at the centre of his learning theory; by learning or conditioning it permits a person to anticipate danger, or other noxious situations. It can be detached from its original association with a painful stimulus and, by secondary learning, become attached to new situations. In this way it is a powerful tool and source of motivation. On the other hand, the learning theorists have demonstrated that fear-provoked behaviour is often very resistant to change, even when the painful stimuli are no longer present (e.g. electric shock). Such evidence sheds light on the persistence of human behaviour which is quite obviously maladaptive: it was probably once successful in reducing fear.

Mowrer was influenced in his views by FREUD's theory of anxiety (synonymous here with fear) (FREUD, 1936, 1949). For FREUD, anxiety was central; it was the warning signal that there was danger for the individual from the outside *real* world. FREUD distinguished between real, neurotic, and moral anxiety. In the last analysis all anxiety stems from reality, and FREUD's distinction rests on the psychic media by which it is experienced, but it does have value in distinguishing between fear of the known danger (real anxiety) and fear of the unknown danger (neurotic and moral anxiety). The individual must take action to reduce anxiety since it is painful to him. If, however, he does not know the source of his anxiety, he can only reduce it by one of the mechanisms we have already discussed — repression, rationalization, etc. It is in this sense that one can say that the reactions of many people to cancer symptoms are neurotic; they are reacting not to the physical symptoms themselves, but to the neurotic and moral anxiety created by false ideas about having cancer. It is with such "unreasonable" and often excessive fear that health-educators and doctors may have to contend.

Without going too deeply into the arguments in support of various lists of basic motives, it is clear that many important "motives" are probably derived, or receive their motive power, from underlying fear.

It is important to stress that we are dealing with fear almost to the exclusion of other basic emotions and motives, not because it is the only or most effective one, but (a) because of its crucial role in matters concerning health, (b) because it is often an easy way to motivate people (but not necessarily to make them act!), and (c) because of its peculiar and often contrary effects. From the earlier discussion of the mechanisms used to defend against anxiety, it is clear that the use of fear as a motivator is quite likely to result in failure if the fear is unavoidable or irreducible by normal means, that is, if all attempts to leave the situation are frustrated and the only possible exits are fear-associated. No-one would deny that fear is a necessary source of adaptive behaviour, particularly when an isolated and immediate action is desired (LEVENTHAL and KAFES, 1963), but studies in several areas of psychology demonstrate its limitations:

Psychologists, in their experiments with animals, have shown that if fear is too intense it is likely to impede rather than assist performance. A "law" (quite old for psychology) was stated by YERKES and DODSON in 1908, indicating a relationship between task-difficulty and optimal level of motivation. *Activation Theorists,* who see motivation in terms of intensity of activation or arousal, have demonstrated that as arousal (e. g. due to "fear") increases, so does efficiency, until an optimal or best point is reached, following which there is a decline in efficiency as arousal continues to increase. (DUFFY, 1932, 1957, 1962).

Communication Studies carried out at Yale (HOVLAND *et al.*, 1953) demonstrated the inefficacy of the use of fear appeals; a more recent study (LEVENTHAL and KAFES, 1963) using antismoking communications has produced further support for this finding. They found that acceptance of a communication increases as the amount of fear increases up to an optimal point, after which acceptance declines as fear increases. We shall deal with this more fully when considering the effects of communications on the changing of attitudes (see page 46 below).

Some workers have suggested (see p. 10 for discussion) that people delayed not out of ignorance of the facts, but out of fear. There is also direct evidence from Russia (ORLOVSKY, 1957) that the use of fear as the stimulus in cancer compaigns was a failure and in consequence was abandoned (see also LA POINTE *et al.*, 1959). The importance of these considerations for health educators is summarized in *Health Education Monographs* No. 6. by R. S. LAZARUS (1959).

Before leaving the topic of fear a word or two must be said about how it is learned. How does a person come to fear a particular thing, or object, or experience? It may be as a result of personal experience, or via the usual channels of communication that exist in any society or culture, or by association with something that is already feared. In other words, we come to fear something according to the usual principles of learning (see the later section on "learning", page 35).

There are many motivating drives apart from that of fear, which are evident in adult behaviour. Some of these, such as hope, can be seen in relation to fear, or as functioning in an inverse way. There has been a growing realization among psychologists, especially those influenced by psychoanalysis, that man develops beyond the stage at which he is at the mercy of his instincts, and past the stage where he is concerned with bringing them into line with reality; his control increases to the point at which he can take an autonomous, dynamic, and creative stand in respect to his environment and himself. Two forms of motivation which have been the concern of social psychologists to an increasing extent are man's desire to be with other people physically, psychologically, and socially (affiliation motivation), and secondly the level of achievement or success that a person requires of himself (achievement motivation).

Finally, and most important of all, the health educator should not become disconcerted because people do not react in the way we (or any other "reasonable" person) would expect in a particular situation. Men react according to the way *they* see the situation, how it affects *them, their* values and possessions, and not according to the logic of the doctor, the lawyer, or even the health educator.

Helpful references for studies of motivation are COFER and APPLEY's (1964) excellent book *Motivation: Theory and Research,* ATKINSON's *An Introduction to Motivation* (1964), also the reviews by MOWRER, COFER, and IRWIN in *The Annual Review of Psychology* for the years 1952, 1959 and 1961, respectively. McCLELLAND's *Studies in Motivation* (1955) is a useful and interesting collection of readings. For a fuller coverage of the field with contributions from almost every area, the *Nebraska Symposium* edited by M. R. JONES has appeared every year since 1953 (COFER 1957 surveys the first five of these). For a brief, sound and readily understandable book on this subject the reader may consult MURRAY (1964).

References: Motivation

AITKEN-SWAN, J., and EASSON, E. C. (1959). Reactions of cancer patients on being told their diagnosis *Brit. med. J.* (i), 779.

ATKINSON, J. W. (1964). *An introduction to motivation*. Princeton. N. J.: Van Nostrand.

COFER, C. N. (1959). Motivation. *Ann. Rev. Psychol.* 10, 173.

COFER, C. N., and APPLEY, M. H. (1964). *Motivation: Theory and research*. New York: John Wiley & Sons.

DOLLARD, J., and MILLER, N. E. (1950). *Personality and Psychotherapy: An analysis in terms of learning, thinking, and culture*, New York: McGraw-Hill.

DUFFY, E. (1932). The relation between muscular tension and quality of performance. *Amer. J. Psychol.* 44, 535.

DUFFY, E. (1957). The psychological significance of the concept of 'Arousal' or Activation. *Psychol. Rev.* 64, 265.

DUFFY, E. (1962). *Activation and behavior*, New York: John Wiley & Sons.

FREUD, A. (1937). *The ego and the mechanisms of defence*. London: Hogarth.

FREUD, S. (1936). *The problem of anxiety*, New York: W. W. Norton.

FREUD, S. (1949). *An outline of psychoanalysis*, New York: W. W. Norton.

HOVLAND, C., JANIS, I. L., and KELLEY, H. H. (1953). *Communication and persuasion*, New Haven: Yale University Press.

IRWIN, F. W. (1961). Motivation and performance. *Ann. Rev. Psychol.* 12, 217.

JANIS, I. L., and LEVENTHAL, H. (1966). Psychological aspects of physical illness and hospital care. In: *Handbook of clinical psychology*, ed. by B. WOLLMAN New York: McGraw-Hill Book Co.

A thoughtful review which is general in application, but contains much of interest to those whose particular interest is in cancer. Discussion of fear, anxiety and worry (before, during and after treatment) is very stimulating, since it takes account of both the 'desirable' and 'undesirable' effects on behaviour.

JONES, M. R. (Ed.) (1953—). *Nebraska symposium on motivation*, Lincoln: University of Nebraska Press.

LA POINTE, J. L., WITTKOWER, E. D., and LOUGHEED, M. N. (1959). The psychiatric evaluation of the effect of cancer education on the lay public. *Cancer* (Philad.) 12, 1200.

LAZARUS, R. S. (1959). Motivation — some basic psychological issues. *Health Education Monographs* No 6.

LEEPER, R. W. (1943). *Lewin's Topographical and vector psychology: A digest and a critique*. Eugene: University Oregon Press.

LEVENTHAL, H., and KAFES, P. N. (1963). The effectiveness of fear-arousing movies in motivating preventive health measures. *N. Y. St. J. med.* 63, 867.

LEWIN, K. (1931). Environmental forces in child behavior and development. In: *A handbook of child psychology*, ed. by C. MURCHISON. Worcester, Mass.: Clark University Press.

LEWIN, K. (1935). *A dynamic theory of personality: Selected papers*. New York: McGraw-Hill Book Co.

LEWIN, K. (1938). *The conceptual representation and the measurement of psychological forces*, Durham, N. C.: Duke University Press.

McCLELLAND, D. C. (Ed.) (1955). *Studies in motivation*, New York: Appleton-Century-Crofts.

MAIER, N. R. F. (1949). *Frustration: The study of behaviour without a goal.* New York: McGraw-Hill.

MAIER, N. R. F. (1956). Frustration theory: Restatement and extension. *Psychol. Rev.* 63, 370.

MILLER, N. E. (1944). Experimental studies of conflict. In: *Personality and the behavior disorders,* ed. by J. Mc V. HUNT. New York: Ronald Press.

MILLER, N. E. (1951). Learnable drives and rewards. In: *Handbook of experimental psychology,* ed. by S. S. STEVENS, New York: John Wiley & Sons.

MOWRER, O. H. (1952). "Motivation". *Ann. Rev. Psychol.* 3, 419.

MOWRER, O. H. (1960a). *Learning theory and behavior. New York: John Wiley & Sons.*

MOWRER, O. H. (1960b). *Learning theory*

and the symbolic processes. New York: John Wiley & Sons.

MURRAY, E. J. (1964). *Motivation and emotion,* Englewood Cliffs, N. J.: Prentice Hall.

ORLOVSKY, L. V. (1957). Anti-cancer propaganda. In: *Methodological manual of anti-cancer propaganda,* ed. by N. N. BLOKHIN, 4th. ed. Moscow: Institute of Health Education. (Russian Text).

PAVLOV, I. P. (1927). *Conditioned reflexes.* London: Oxford University Press: Humphrey Milford.

SUTHERLAND, A. M. (1959). Psychological impact of cancer and its therapy. In: *Cancer,* ed. by R. W. RAVEN, vol. 6. London: Butterworth & Co.

WATERS, R. H., RETHLINGSHAFER, D. A., and CALDWELL, W. E. (Eds.) (1960). *Principles of comparative psychology,* New York: McGraw-Hill Book Co.

7. Perception

Perception refers to the way sensory experiences are assimilated and understood by the individual. BERELSON and STEINER describe it as "the more complex process than sensations by which people select, organize, and interpret sensory stimulation into a meaningful and coherent picture of the world". (BERELSON and STEINER, 1964, p. 88).

The main aspect of perception to be dealt with here is that there is no one-to-one correspondence between what the *senses* experience as a result of stimulation and what the *person* experiences. Our present task is to examine some of the factors which bear on this.

The first thing involved in perception is the manner in which the person *attends* to his environment. But attention itself is subject to a number of factors. Since it is dependent, to a certain extent, on the senses and supporting bodily functions, it will necessarily be subject to the normal laws of *fatigue* — i. e. attention will be less when one is physically tired, or when one has been at the task a long time,

though length of time is not all that is involved. Interest is the most obvious factor involved in how long we persist in a task and how hard we try at it. The interest involved in attention or vigilance can be affected by whether or not we feel that we may benefit by it, or by our being emotionally involved in it (e. g. because it affects something we value), or by there being a need that may be fulfilled by it — which all boils down to its being sufficiently important to us. A third factor involved in strength of attention is our *expectation* or *anticipation* that a particular event will take place. This factor is synomymous with the concept of "set"; there will be a predisposition to perceive things in a fixed (or set) way under the influence of, for instance, bias, attitudes, prejudice and special interests. This has been discussed by several authors in different terminology, e. g. schema (BARTLETT, 1932), assumptions (AMES, 1955), hypotheses (BRUNER, 1951). Expectation, however, has two sides to it: it will sometimes enable us to observe something which we would otherwise miss (e. g. we expect to see an unpleasant look on our enemy's face), but it also makes a novelty more noticeable (e. g. a fair Latin, or a dark Anglo-Saxon). The fourth and final factor influencing attention is the strength and other characteristics of the *sensory input* from the stimulus; a powerful stimulus will attract our attention more readily.

Closely related to attention is *selection:* what the individual selects from the innumerable bits of information he receives about his environment *via* his senses. Obviously he cannot attend to all his physical and social surroundings at once, hence the functioning of attention as outlined above. Further selection is made along similar lines, until finally only a relatively small area of the whole possible perceptional field reaches the person. Through the influence of motives, interests, values, emotions, etc., selection is made of the relevant objects; (see JENKIN 1957); defences are put up to prevent the perception of unpleasant or potentially disturbing or irrelevant objects. (See BRUNER and POSTMAN, 1947; McGINNIES, 1949; BROWN 1961). There is abundant evidence that these perceptual processes affect the perceived characteristics of the object. Thus BRUNER and POSTMAN (1948) demonstrated that positive and negative values (of a dollar sign and a swastika) led to the subject's overestimating the size of the plastic discs on which these were drawn as compared with a neutral (geometric) sign. (see, also LAMBERT *et al.,* 1949). POSTMAN *et al.* (1948) demonstrated that personal value-systems (e. g. religious, economic) can affect one's perception and memory (cf. also POSTMAN and SCHNEIDER 1955). McCLELLAND and ATKINSON (1948) have shown the effects of hunger on the perception of volunteers: food-related objects (e. g. fork, table) increased in frequency (up to a point) when

the subjects were asked to relate what they perceived, when in fact nothing was there. POSTMAN and BRUNER (1948) have shown the effect of stress on perception, resulting in a kind of perceptual recklessness. ATKINSON and his co-workers have shown that motivation to achievement (i. e. to succeed) can affect recall of an unfinished task (ATKINSON, 1955). There is also evidence about the effect that racial attitudes and one's own colour can have on perception. (SEELMAN, 1940; MARKS, 1943). The processes of perception will have similar effects on what is learned and what is remembered.

It is important to note that perception is amenable to training. Examples of this in everyday experience are not hard to find: the doctor examining a slide under a microscope or an x-ray; the farmer noticing the finer points in his animal's condition, breast self-examination for cancer symptoms. There is also experimental evidence for this from HAGGARD and ROSE (1944), and SCHAFER and MURPHY (1943) among others. Much of the research into the discrimination of different stimuli and learning to discriminate between different stimuli and patterns of stimuli is in fact research into perception. (see WOODWORTH and SCHLOSBERG, 1955, p. 582 ff.; OSGOOD, 1953, p. 350 ff.). A third source of evidence regarding the element of learning in perception is to be found in the many social, cultural and anthropological studies of attitudes. (e. g. PAUL, 1955) and prejudices (APPLE, 1960; HURLOCK, 1964; RAAB and LIPSET, 1959; SHERIF, 1935; also the many studies on social conformity.) As a result of experiments, especially with visual objects, a law of perception has been proposed which states that, particularly where there is ambiguity in the stimuli, one will organize what one sees according to one's expectations and needs; that the part will be seen in relation to the whole, that is, in context; and there will be a tendency to homogeneity, so that there will be symmetry, regularity and simplicity of perception.

Extending these laws to the non-sensory, we can see that they have obvious application to the organization of information, to memory, (see BARTLETT, 1932), and to such things as the composition and functioning of social groups. Regarding the effect that perception has on the reception and acceptance of communication, we shall have more to say later. Man's activities in his society, and even the society itself, are, to a large extent, governed by the way he perceives his environment. We follow men we perceive to possess the qualities we expect in a leader, and whom we perceive to promise satisfaction of our needs. We listen to men we perceive to possess the necessary qualifications of reliability, and who will not contradict what we hold strongly. We associate with men we perceive are like ourselves, satisfy our desire for comradeship, etc. We blame men we perceive to be the cause of harm to us. For an extensive consideration of this we refer the reader to *Person Perception and Interpersonal Behaviour*, edited by TAGIURI and PETRULLO (1958). (See also BRUNER and TAGIURI, 1954; TAGIURI et al., 1958; JONES and deCHARMS 1958.) WOODWORTH (1958) places great stress on the interaction between man and his environment, and emphasises the function of perception in man's "dealing with the environment". [See KUTNER (1958) for social perception in the patient-surgeon relationship.]

The usefulness of these findings has been greatly increased by recent evidence for the existence of a relationship between personality and perception. If it is true that certain types of people perceive in a particular way, or even that people tend to perceive in a fairly consistent way, then our powers of prediction of people's behaviour are enormously increased. (See ALLPORT, 1958; BLAKE and RAMSEY, 1951; WITKIN et al., 1954.)

For the health-educator, the way a person or potential patient perceives the educator, doctor, hospital, illness, etc., is of crucial importance. (See Chapter Five on this subject). The factors of experience, learning, and expectations are important, for example, in the current situation, where the public is aware mainly of those cancer cases that are fatal.

For a comprehensive review of the theories of perception and research in this field, the reader is referred to F. H. ALLPORT's book, *Theories of Perception and the Concept of Structure* (1955). For a consideration of the research with less emphasis on theory he is referred to VERNON (1952). OSGOOD (1953) has an excellent section (pp. 191—298) covering all aspects of perception and some of the theoretical problems involved. Various sections of BERELSON and STEINER (1964) give useful summaries in the different areas of psychology. A useful and yet not too advanced book is ABERCROMBIE's *The Anatomy of Judgment* (1960). A lecture given by G. W. ALLPORT to health educators on "Perception and Public Health" is issued as one of the *Health Education Monographs* (1958). HOCHBERG (1964) deals with perception briefly, simply and interestingly.

References: Perception

ABERCROMBIE, M. L. J. (1960). *The anatomy of judgment*. London: Hutchinson.

ALLPORT, F. H. (1955). *Theories of perception and the concept of structure*. New York: John Wiley & Sons.

ALLPORT, G. W. (1958). Perception and public health. *Health Education Monographs*, No 2.

AMES, A. (1955). *An interpretative manual for the demonstrations in the psychology research centre*. Princeton: Princeton University Press.

APPLE, D. (1960). *Sociological studies of health and sickness*, New York: McGraw-Hill Book Co.

ATKINSON, J. N. (1955). The achievement motive and recall of interrupted and completed tasks. In: *Studies in motivation*, ed. by D. C. McCLELLAND. New York: Appleton-Century-Crofts.

BARTLETT, F. C. (1932). *Remembering*. Cambridge: Cambridge University Press.

BERELSON, B., and STEINER, G. A. (1964). *Human behavior: An inventory of scientific findings*. New York: Harcourt, Brace & World.

BLAKE, R. R., and RAMSEY, G. V. (Eds.) (1951). *Perception: An approach to personality*. New York: Ronald Press.

BROWN, W. (1961). Conceptions of perceptual defence. *Brit. J. Psych. Monograph*. 35.

BRUNER, J. S. (1951). Personality dynamics and the process of perceiving. In: *Perception: An approach to personality*, ed. by R. R. BLAKE and G. V. RAMSEY. New York: Ronald Press.

BRUNER, J. S., and POSTMAN, L. (1947). Emotional selectivity in perception and reaction. *J. Personality* 16, 69.

BRUNER, J. S., and POSTMAN, L. (1948). Symbolic value as an organizing factor in perception. *J. Soc. Psychol.* 27, 203.

BRUNER, J. S., and TAGIURI, R. (1954). The perception of people. In: *Handbook of social psychology*, ed. by G. LINDZEY, vol. II. Cambridge (Mass.): Addison-Wesley.

HAGGARD, E. A., and ROSE, G. J. (1944). Some effects of mental set and active participation in the conditioning of the autokinetic phenomenon. *J. Exp. Psychol.* 34, 45.

HOCHBERG, J. E. (1964). *Perception*, Englewood Cliffs, N. J.: Prentice-Hall.

HURLOCK, E. B. (1964). *Child development*. New York: McGraw-Hill Book Co.

JENKIN, N. (1957). Affective processes in perception. *Psychol. Bull.* 54, 100.

JONES, E. E., and DE CHARMS, R. (1958). Changes in social perception as a function of the personal relevance of behaviour. In: *Readings in social psychology*, ed. by E. E. MACCOBY et al. New York: Holt, Rinehart & Winston.

KUTNER, B. (1958). Surgeons and their patients: A Study in social perception. In: *Patients, physicians and illness*, ed. by E. G. JACO. Glencoe, Ill.: Free Press.

LAMBERT, W. W., SOLOMON, R. L., and WATSON, P. D. (1949). Reinforcement and extinction as factors in size estimation. *J. exp. Psych.* 39, 637.

MARKS, E. S. (1943). Skin color judgments of negro college students. *J. abnorm. soc. psychol.* 38, 370.

McCLELLAND, D. C., and ATKINSON, J. W. (1948). The projective expression of needs: 1. The effect of different intensities of the hunger drive on perception. *J. Psychol.* (Provincetown) 25, 205.

McGINNIES, E. (1949). Emotionality and perceptual defense. *Psychol. Rev.* 56, 244.

OSGOOD, C. E. (1953). *Method and theory in experimental psychology*. New York: Oxford University Press.

PAUL, B. (Ed.) (1955). *Health, culture, and community*. New York: Russell Sage Foundation.

POSTMAN, L., and BRUNER, J. S. (1948). Perception under stress. *Psychol. Rev.* 55, 314.

POSTMAN, L., BRUNER, J. S., and McGINNIES, E. (1948). Personal values as selective factors in perception. *J. abnorm. soc. Psychol.* 43, 142.

POSTMAN, L., and SCHNEIDER, B. H. (1955). Personal values, visual recognition, and recall. In: *Studies in motivation*, ed. by D. C. McCLELLAND. New York: Appleton-Century-Crofts.

RAAB, E., and LIPSET, S. M. (1959). *Prejudice and society*. New York: Anti-Defamation League of B'nai B'rith.

SCHAFER, R., and MURPHY, G. (1943). The role of antism in a visual figure-ground relationship. *J. exp. Psychol.* **32**, 335.

SEELMAN, V. (1940). The influence of attitude upon the remembering of pictorial material. *Arch. Psych.* No **258**.

SHERIF, M. (1935). A study of some social factors in perception. *Arch. Psych.* No **187**.

TAGIURI, R., BRUNER, J. S., and BLAKE, R. R. (1958). On the relation between feelings and perception of feelings among members of small groups. In: *Readings in social psychology*, ed. by E. E. MACCOBY *et al.* New York: Holt, Rinehart & Winston.

TAGIURI, R., and PETRULLO, L. (Eds.) (1958). *Person perception and interpersonal behavior.* Stanford: Stanford University Press.

VERNON, M. D. (1952). *A further study of visual perception.* Cambridge: Cambridge University Press.

WITKIN, H. A., LEWIS, H. B., HERTZMAN, M., MACHOVER, K., BRETNALL MEISSNER, P., and WAPNER, S. (1954). *Personality through perception.* New York: Harper.

WOODWORTH, R. S. (1958). *Dynamics of behaviour.* London: Methuen & Co.

WOODWORTH, R. S., and SCHLOSBERG, H. (1955). *Experimental psychology.* London: Methuen & Co.

8. Learning

The expression "learning theory" will be used here to refer loosely to those parts of psychology that deal with the way in which individuals learn. There have been relatively few attempts to draw conclusions from this field of study and apply them to health education. Learning theory, though a specialised field in itself, has never really surmounted the hurdle presented by the sheer complexity of human behaviour. As a result, it has tried to simplify its object of study by using lower animal species and also by theoretically isolating the elements of behaviour (e. g. incentive, drive, habit, inhibition, etc.). Little can therefore be validly extrapolated for application to human behaviour. But there are two ways in which learning theory may be of assistance. We may be able to glean a few indications or clues to guide us to the human situation. Secondly, we can examine the one area in which human subjects have been studied extensively — the process of remembering.

One of the corner-stones of all learning theories has been the concept of reinforcement, and though psychologists differ in their views about the nature of reinforcement, it is one of the most prominent aspects of learning in everyday life. Any attempt to define "reinforcement" will depend on whether one takes a pragmatic or a hedonistic point of view. From the pragmatic viewpoint, reinforcement refers to *anything* that increases the probability of a certain action being performed. From the hedonistic viewpoint, reinforcement is seen solely in terms of pleasure and pain, pleasure increasing (reinforcing) the likelihood that an action will be performed, and pain reducing it (negatively reinforcing). For our present purposes a combination of both is probably most useful. People are more likely to do things that are pleasurable and avoid those that are painful; but one must remember that, although some things are generally agreed to be pleasurable or painful, there are many occasions on which more than one interpretation is possible, and it then becomes a personal, subjective matter. Prior study is, then, required to discover just what people regard as pleasurable and what as painful, and to what extent they do so. Thus, going to see the doctor may be pleasurable (or rewarding) for some individuals, classes of individuals, or sections of society, but painful (or punishing) for others. There are, for instance, some societies — such as peasant communities in Greece — which regard seeking medical advice as a sign of weakness; yet some tribal societies in Africa regard prompt care of the breadwinner as an urgent and vital duty. The two norms of behaviour would colour the views of individuals in those communities regarding what constitutes rewarding or punishing activity. Psychologists usually talk in terms of reward and punishment. Bearing in mind what we have said above, these two terms may, with care, be used as alternatives for pleasure and pain.

Ignoring variations in the points of view of different psychologists concerning the definition of 'reinforcement' and the part it plays in learning, one can say that reward and punishment have their own characteristic effects in the learning situation. Careful consideration should be given to what behaviour one wishes to produce. Taking a simple situation of doing or not doing a certain action which we will call A, the aims of the educator can be (i) Not to do A — and, by inference, doing anything else but A; or (ii) not to do A but to do B or (iii) to do A. There are several possible combinations of reward and/or punishment which may be used to achieve (i), (ii) or (iii). For (i) it should be sufficient merely to punish the doing of A. (ii) can be achieved by making a reward attached to the performance of B sufficiently attractive to exclude that of A; it may be necessary, though, to punish any attempt at A. For (iii) one must either reward A, or exclude by means of punishment all other alternatives. It must be pointed out, however, that the above is one of the simplest of situations. There will usually be more than two possible courses of action, and each one will be more *or* less attractive or repulsive. Furthermore, the importance of the strength of the punishment must be stressed, for, if it is too great, there is a possibility that it will have a paralysing effect, and (in (ii) for example) the subject when punished for doing A will "freeze" and be unable to follow the alternative course of action, B. Without taking sides with one theory or another, this is the effect that has been found both in experiments by learning theorists and also in communication studies which use fear as a motivator.

MOWRER calls attention to the different consequences of the use of the two types of reinforcement. Discussing the effect of what he calls danger signals [1] (stimuli, objects, or situations repeatedly associated with punishment) he says "a teacher (or any other person) who is constantly emitting danger signals will tend to drive students *away* from her (and from the school situation in general), whereas a teacher who emits safety signals and promises (which are confirmed tends to *attract* them. And this is important educationally" (MOWRER, 1960).

An important experimental finding supports what one would expect from common sense; punishment that is *avoidable* is much more effective than that which is *unavoidable*. This is important in everyday life, in which going to the doctor when something serious is suspected may seem to involve unavoidable punishment if the patient believes that nothing can be done, or knows that treatment will be long or painful. There is also evidence that subjects prefer a situation in which there is a warning signal of danger that permits avoiding action. It is likely that when punishment is unavoidable other defences will be attempted. In the case of human beings these will often be mental

---

[1] It should be noted that Mowrer's use of the term "danger signals" is in no sense synonymous with the use of the same term in the public education programmes of the American and Canadian Cancer Societies.

defences, such as denial or withdrawal. (See page 26 of this work.)

Just as certain stimuli obtain their significance from association with punishment, others associated with reward or the avoidance of punishment can act as safety signals, or can in themselves be reinforcing by means of what is termed "secondary reinforcement". This is a crucial concept in all learning theories, if not in all learning, and has been used to explain all sorts of anomalies.

One of the most important factors in reinforcement is what has been called the "schedule" of reinforcement i.e. how often and when an action is reinforced or punished. There is a great deal of evidence to show that an action that is reinforced intermittently (i.e. not on every occasion) is harder to extinguish than an action reinforced on every occasion. This is possibly due to the effect produced when a person finds that a situation no longer holds true; a single exception can disprove a rule stated as universally true, but will not have such an effect on a rule only claimed to hold in certain cases — hence the inadvisability of making false claims in educating the public, as, for example, giving the impression that all cancers are curable.

The delay between an action and the reward of punishment of that action should, from common-sense and experimental evidence, diminish the power the reinforcement has. Only infrequently in everyday life do all the good and bad results of behaviour follow immediately or even closely after its completion. It is, therefore, a crucial problem in the most significant areas of social learning to bridge the gap between act and consequence. In cancer education an obvious example is the often lengthy time-lag between the first seemingly trivial symptoms that lead to delay in seeing a doctor and the onset of painful or incapacitating symptoms. The problem is even greater when the relationship between act and consequence is further obscured by immediate satisfaction, as in the case of cigarette smoking.

An interesting situation arises when elements of both reward and punishment are present. The individual concerned may either exaggerate the reward of his action (maximize the gain), e. g. by going to the doctor, regardless of his belief that treatment may be painful or financially crippling; or he may play down the punishment aspect (minimize the loss) by staying away and offsetting the danger to his health by his continued freedom from painful treatment and financial loss. It has been suggested that how the individual will assess the situation may well be a question of personality. No one form of education can therefore hope to encompass all the possible variants of human response, and it is important for the educator to be constantly aware of this in designing his programme.

An important aspect of any learning situation is the extent to which the learning is aided or hindered by the similarity of present circumstances and actions to those of previous learning situations. It is evident that when a new response has to be learned there is a problem of habit-breaking. A habit will be more difficult to break the older it is, or the more it has been practised. It will also be difficult to break if the new and old responses are incompatible. It is therefore obvious that a health educator will find great difficulty in changing old-established patterns of behaviour or attitudes when they are incompatible with the new response (e.g. the old habit of denying the existence of an illness and the desired new response of seeking prompt medical care).

The topic of remembering is only one part of the complex field of learning, but in many respects it is the most important aspect of the eductional process. No attempt will be made here to summarize the enormous amount of work that has been done since the earliest days of modern experimental psychology. For an excellent review and critical consideration of this, the reader is referred to chapters 12 and 13 of C. E. Osgood's book *Method and Theory in Experimental Psychology* (1953).

Recognizing that we shall leave ourselves open to the criticism of oversimplification, we nevertheless think it is useful to consider some of the main elements involved in remembering. The first is a short-term temporal factor, which accounts for the build-up and dissipation of inhibition. The inhibition referred to here is the sort that develops throughout the performance of an action or with repeated performance, that is, a type of fatigue. This temporal factor helps to explain the phenomena of the bow-shaped curve of learning, reminiscence, and the superiority of distributed practice. We shall deal only with the last of these phenomena.

Distribution of learning refers to the way in which it is spread out through time. Thus a person learning a list of words must decide (i) how slowly he will read each word, (ii) how many words he will read before taking a rest, and (iii) how many times he will read the entire list before resting. The experimental evidence demonstrates the superiority of distributed learning as opposed to massed learning. In practical terms these results mean that it is advantageous to procede slowly, with pauses sufficient to allow for the dissipation of "fatigue".

The second factor is known as interference. The basis of this is the similarity between (i) elements of the material to be learned e. g. the similarity of words in a list of words, or (ii) the similarity between the learned material and subsequent material. For instance, the learning and remembering of a list of words will suffer more interference if the subject is faced with the highly similar task of learning another list of words than if he is called on to learn the dissimilar task of driving a car. Constant exposure to similar learning tasks accounts for the cumulative loss in retention of material with time.

There are also other factors that both common-sense and experimental evidence tell us must influence learning and remembering. The meaningfulness of material is one such. It is obviously easier to learn ten words which form a meaningful sentence than ten unconnected words. Trite though this statement may seem, it is too often disregarded in preparing material for the general public. It is all too easy for the specialist in medicine or health education to frame his message in the language of his own reference group. Even when a conscious effort is made to avoid mishap, only careful testing of the material will ensure that it conveys the meaning intended without the intrusion of uncomprehended factors. Another such factor is motivation, which plays as large a part in learning as in any other field of human behaviour. We remember better those things in which we are personally involved. The educator must therefore discover and make use, in his educational programme, of the hopes, fears, social norms and existing beliefs of his audience, so that his message will appear to have the most personal appeal possible to the recipient.

Before closing this section, we should mention the important influence that perception may have on the processes of remembering and learning. Perception, as used here, does not refer to the use of the five senses, but to the way in which communications are grasped at the intellectual level. The two forms of perception,

though distinct, are in many ways an-
alagous, and some of the principles derived from the study of sensory perception apply equally to intellectual perception. One of the most important of
these principles is that of "set", which we
have already defined as a predisposition
to perceive things in a fixed (or set) way,
under the influence of, for instance, bias,
attitudes, prejudice, and special interests.
This principle is also included in laws put
forward originally by the Gestalt psychologists, and summed up by the *law of
prägnanz*, according to which "psychological organization will always be as
'good' as prevailing conditions allow". In
simple terms, this means that the way in
which people perceive, receive and organize the information offered will tend
to follow a pattern of symmetry, regularity and simplicity. They tend either to
make communications fit in with what
they already believe, or to complete the
(to them) unfinished picture by a series of
illogical steps, or to simplify the message
to make it more manageable. All these
processes can be a potent mechanism of
distortion, twisting the message the educator *thinks* he has put over into something quite other than he intended. The
same principle also accounts for much of
the change in what is remembered (or
what is forgotten) that occurs over time.

Probably the most complete reviews
of research into the processes of learning
are *Theories of Learning* by E. R. HIL-
GARD (1958), and *Conditioning and
Learning* by E. R. HILGARD and D. G.
MARQUIS, revised and edited by G. A.
KIMBLE (1961). An excellent, brief, and
not too advanced book on the subject is
Learning by S. A. Mednick (1964). The
readers should find useful any of the many
books available on educational psychology; especially recommended is *Educational Psychology* by D. R. GREEN
(1964), (also Cronbach, 1963; Valentine,
1960).

References: Learning

CRONBACH, L. J. (1963). *Educational psychology*. New York: Harcourt, Brace &
World.

GREEN, D. R. (1964). *Educational psychology*. Englewood Cliffs, N. J.:
Prentice — Hall.

HILGARD, E. R. (1958). *Theories of learning*, London: Methuen.

HILGARD, E. R., and MARQUIS, D. G.
(1961). *Conditioning and learning*.
London: Methuen. Rev. and ed. by
G. A. KIMBLE.

MEDNICK, S. A. (1964). *Learning*, Englewood Cliffs, N. J.: Prentice — Hall.

MOWRER, O. H. (1960). *Learning theory
and behavior*. New York: John Wiley & Sons.

OSGOOD, C. E. (1953). *Method and theory in experimental psychology*. New
York: Oxford University Press.

VALENTINE, C. W. (1960). *Psychology
and its bearing on education*, London:
Methuen.

9. Roles

We shall deal later with the functioning of groups. Studies of groups have
importance for many reasons. They are,
first of all, the unit of society in which
all behaviour takes place: men never act
in a vacuum, they are always members
of a number of groups, and their actions
will have an effect on some at least of the
members of some of these groups. Secondly, the attitudes of the individual are to a
great extent derived from, and reinforced
or maintained by, the relevant groups to
which he belongs and with which he interacts. Lastly, we stress the importance

of group-studies because the health educator is so often concerned with influencing the individual through the group (for example, the audience or the discussion-group). In dealing with group-studies we will have cause to mention the effect of a person's status or position in the group on the power the group has over his behaviour and attitudes.

In any group there is an uneven distribution, if not of power, then at least of status or ranking (which can be based on any number of different criteria). There is also a distribution of functions or tasks according to the aims, values and needs of the group. Certain members of the group, therefore, have to perform certain tasks when called upon to do so either formally by the members or rules of the group, or less formally as a consequence of being a member of the group, or possessing the qualities or skills necessary to carry out the task. In this way the group and its members come to *expect* the performance of certain actions by different members. When this happens, the person in question fills a *role* in the group which entails the fulfilling of certain duties by that person in line with the expectations and rights of the group. Roles within a group (e. g. family) are sometimes specified and controlled by the wider cultural environment in which a person exists.

The mere fact that a group expects the holder of a role-position to act in a particular way does not necessarily imply that he will either be aware of this, or that, being aware of it, he will act accordingly. In this case, as in many others, the way a person perceives the role and its associated expectations will be of paramount importance. A distinction must therefore, be made between roles and role-behaviour.

It is not uncommon to find that two individuals occupying similar role-positions will behave in different ways as a result of different interpretations of the duties involved. On the other hand, a role is very often independent of the occupier of the role, since the role can continue to exist in spite of there being a number of different individuals holding the role-position over a period of time, or even if there is no one occupying the role at all. We can say, therefore, that there is a certain continuity associated with a role. Since an individual occupies many positions simultaneously (e. g. father, worker, patient) there will be several expectations to be fulfilled at any one time. Sometimes these expectations will be incompatible with each other or with those of another person; on other occasions confusion will arise from the lack of agreement by members of a group about the expectations of a particular role. In such cases of conflict or confusion a person will have to solve the conflict by the use of one or more of the following: relinquishing one of the roles, redefining the expectations, or limiting the function of the roles so as to ensure a separation of the conflicting roles.

We have been talking about roles in terms of the group. It must be made clear, however, that groups are as diverse in their characteristics as are the forms of interaction and relationships between two or more people. Whenever two or more individuals interact socially there are always a number of expectations (expressed or understood) about the behaviour of the one with respect to the other, and to this extent a person is always occupying some role (e. g. Superior-inferior, older-younger) when he interacts with other people. Roles are thus the link between an individual and society.

The lesson from all this for the health-educator is that a person never acts in isolation but is always a member of a group, whether it be a formally constructed one or merely the informal interaction between two people (e. g. health educator and recipient).

The educator should ask himself what the recipient of his communication expects of him in the role of health-educator, doctor or any other role he might *be seen* to occupy. The recipient's expectations about his own behaviour as a result of being in the role of recipient, patient, pupil, etc., must also be examined.

Of perhaps greatest use to the educator in the planning of a health education programme is a clear perception of the structure of the society or community in which he is working. By means of an examination of the roles filled by various members of the society, one can identify the key positions at which to direct one's campaign. Such positions are usually filled by those occupying the roles of leaders in the community, whether it be in terms of economics, religion, scholarship, government or any other criterion of status and leadership. This analysis must be made (not necessarily academically, but at least superficially) down through the entire social structure. All the role-positions an individual holds and the role-expectations that go with them (e. g. work, family, government) will have an effect on his behaviour, including that associated with his health. (See Chapter Five on the "sick role"). Such an analysis is even more necessary, since, when working with a society or part of a society with which one is not familiar, one can never presume that positions in the different societies, or even in different parts of the same society, are similar in the duties, rights, and expectations that go with them.

For works on the subject of roles the reader is referred especially to L. R. SARBIN's review in Lindzey (1954), also relevant chapters in *Human Society* by K. DAVIS (1949), and in *Sociological Theory and Social Structure* by R. K. MERTON (1957). NADEL's *The Theory of Social Structure* (1957), NEIMAN and HUGHES's "The Problem of the Concept of Role — a Re-Survey of the Literature" (1951), and PARSON's *The Social System* (1952) should also be consulted.

References: Roles

DAVIS, K. (1949). *Human society*. New York: MacMillan.

MERTON, R. K. (1957). *Social theory and social structure*. Glencoe (Ill.): Free Press.

NADEL, S. F. (1957). *The theory of social structure*. Glencoe (Ill.): Free Press.

NEIMAN, L. J., and HUGHES, J. W. (1951). The Problem of the concept of role: a re-survey of the literature. *Social Forces*, 30, 141.

PARSONS, T. (1952). *The social system*. London: Tavistock.

SARBIN, L. R. (1954). Role theory. In: *Handbook of social psychology*, vol. 1, ed. by G. LINDZEY. Cambridge (Mass).: Addison — Wesley.

Attitudes and Communication

10. Attitudes; Definition and Theory

In the first chapters of this work we presented evidence to show that many people react to the idea of cancer in a largely negative and unwarranted manner. This is only one example of what is commonly termed an attitude. Other examples abound: racial prejudice, political and religious attitudes, etc. Before any attempt can be made to change a person's attitudes, as clear an idea as possible is required of what an attitude consists of. Although there is no unanimity among psychologists on this point, we shall attempt to outline those points on which agreement exists.

First of all, attitude is not a tangible or even an observable thing; it is, rather, a concept used to describe something that is inferred from observable behaviour. The element common to nearly all definitions of an attitude is the consistency in the way a person acts when confronted with a particular object or class of objects (persons or ideas). Observation must be made of a representative sample of behaviour; that is to say, the observations must be spread over a period of time, on a number of occasions, and in relation to several members of the same class of objects, if generalization of one's findings is to be made to a whole class of objects. So, for example, we judge a person's racial attitudes from observing his behaviour on several occasions when he meets individuals of a different race, and from seeing if he behaves in a consistently negative (or positive) manner to people of one racial group as compared with those of another.

The concept of "attitude" is often rendered vague by failure to define its meaning. It should be possible, however, to eliminate much of this vagueness by using behaviour as the criterion. To make an accurate assessment of behaviour is no easy matter, but it is certainly a safer guide to attitudes than the verbal evidence of interested parties. Attitude scales and other forms of attitude measurement are only valid to the extent that they agree with observed behaviour.

Given a broad description of attitudes, we may now ask: of what is an attitude constituted? Theoreticians in this field have distinguished cognitive, affective (emotional), and behavioural components of attitudes (e. g. Katz, 1960).

The supposed presence or absence of these, their interrelations, and the emphasis placed on any of them, differentiate the theories of attitudes and attitude-change.

A governing principle behind several of the theoretical approaches is that whenever there exists an inconsistency between the elements of an attitude, or between a number of attitudes, there is a natural tendency to remove the inconsistency. An example of inconsistency between the elements of an attitude is the conflict between what people know about the dangers of cigarette smoking and their persistence in the habit. Another example is the discrepancy between the good one *knows* about a person and the ill-feeling one has for him (the basis of much prejudice). An example of the inconsistency between two attitudes is the coexistence in one individual of belief in universal suffrage alongside an opposition to votes for a particular section of the community.

How inconsistency is removed will depend on the situation, the attitudes involved, and the individual concerned, his personality etc. A possible solution will be to bring one of the inconsistent elements or attitudes in line with the other. Sometimes this will be done in the most reasonable way, resulting in the individual doing what he knows is best (e. g. by not smoking, or by acting without bias in agreeing to votes for everyone). Such a solution of inconsistency is, unhappily, more of an ideal than a fact. One does not have to look far for examples of irrational solutions. We make frequent use of the defence-mechanisms of repression, rationalization, projection etc. (see page 51 *et seq.* of this work) to eliminate the conflict. A typical example is to argue away or repress the evidence against cigarette smoking (See FEATHER, 1963). Alternatively, the wrong element is sometimes brought into line with the other, as when someone distorts what he knows about another person to lend support to his hostile feelings towards that person. Another example of this, from the field of health education, is provided by people who quote examples of fatal cases of cancer in support of their view that all cancers are inevitably fatal, ignoring the many cases where a successful cure is achieved.

Theories that postulate a principle of the sort outlined above are:

1. Cognitive Dissonance (FESTINGER, 1957, 1964; BREHM and COHEN, 1962).

2. Principle of Congruity (OSGOOD, 1960; OSGOOD *et al*; 1957).

3. Principle of Balance (CARTWRIGHT and HARARY, 1956; HEIDER, 1946, 1958; McGUIRE, 1960; ROSENBERG, 1960, 1965).

4. Strain to Symmetry (NEWCOMB, 1953, 1956).

5. Structural Balance Model (FEATHER, 1964.

6. Homeostatic Theory of Attitude Change (MACCOBY and MACCOBY, 1961).

7. Cognitive Summation Theory (FISHBEIN, 1963; FISHBEIN and HUNTER, 1964).

The listing of the theories in this way should not lead the reader to underestimate the theoretical differences involved. But, on the other hand, it seems safe to say that they are to a great extent complementary, and all have implications for the use of communications in the changing of attitudes. They emphasize the ways in which such communications (e. g. health education programmes) can lead to discrepancies between attitudes, and between elements of an attitude.

They also suggest possible measures that may be taken, whether rational or irrational, to resolve these discrepancies.

If the reader now sees an attitude as a concept much less simple than was previously imagined, this is perhaps a good thing. An attitude is not something that can be easily manipulated and dealt with in isolation. Attitudes, as KATZ (1960) has stressed, serve a purpose in the general complexity of the needs of individuals. Thus, when people have negative attitudes to cancer, the educator must be aware of all their needs (e. g. to preserve life, to protect the family and possessions, etc.) before venturing on any attempt to alter those attitudes.

Worthy of special mention is the research that has been carried out under the Yale Communication and Attitude Change Program. This research has incorporated much of the underlying theory alluded to in this section, and has involved a systematic study of the many factors involved in the use of communications for the changing of attitudes. The main findings are summarized in the next chapter. (See HOVLAND *et al*; 1953; HOVLAND and JANIS, 1959; ROSENBERG *et al*; 1960; SHERIF and HOVLAND, 1961; see also SHERIF *et al*; 1965).

The reader is referred to the following useful publications on the theory of attitudes: *Attitude Change and Social Influence* by A. R. COHEN (1964), B. F. GREEN's chapter on "Attitude Measurement" in G. LINDZEY's *Handbook of Social Psychology* (1954), and the special issue of the *Public Opinion Quarterly* (1960) on "Attitude Change" edited by D. KATZ.

References: Attitudes: definition and theory

BREHM, J. W., and COHEN, A. R. (1962). *Explorations in cognitive dissonance*, New York: John Wiley & Sons.

CARTWRIGHT, D., and HARARY, F. (1956). Structural balance: generalization of HEIDER's theory. *Psychol. Rev.* 63, 277.

COHEN, A. R. (1964). *Attitude change and social influence*, New York: Basic Books.

FEATHER, N. T. (1963). Cognitive dissonance, sensitivity, and evaluation. *J. abnorm. soc. Psychol.* 66, 157.

FEATHER, N. T. (1964). A structural balance model of communication effects. *Psychol. Rev.* 71, 291.

FESTINGER L. (1957). *A theory of cognitive dissonance.* Evanston (Ill.): Row, Peterson. (Stanford: Stanford University Press 1962).

FESTINGER L. (1964). *Conflict, decision and dissonance*, London: Tavistock.

FISHBEIN, M. (1963). An investigation of the relationships between beliefs about an object and the attitude toward that object. *Hum. Relat.* 16, 233.

FISHBEIN, M., and HUNTER, R. (1964). Summation versus balance in attitude organization and change. *J. abnor. soc. Psychol.* 69, 505.

GREEN, B. F. (1964). Attitude measurement. In: *Handbook of social psychology*, volume 1. ed. by G. LINDZEY. Cambridge (Mass.): Addison-Wesley.

HEIDER, F. (1946). Attitudes and cognitive organization. *J. Psychol.* 21, 107.

HEIDER, F. (1958). *The psychology of interpersonal relations.* New York: John Wiley & Sons.

HOVLAND C. I. (Ed.) (1957). *The order of presentation in persuasion.* New Haven (Conn.): Yale University Press.

HOVLAND, C. I., and JANIS, I. L. (Eds.) (1959). *Personality and persuasibility.* New Haven (Conn.) Yale University Press.

HOVLAND, C. I. JANIS, I. L., and KELLEY, H. H. (1953). *Communication and persuasion*, New Haven (Conn.): Yale University Press.

KATZ, D. (1960). The functional approach to the study of attitudes. *Public Opinion Quart.* 24, 163.

MACCOBY, N., and MACCOBY, E. E. (1961). Homeostatic theory in attitude change. *Public Opinion Quart.* 25, 538.

McGUIRE, W. J. (1960). A syllogistic analysis of cognitive relationships. In: *Attitude organisation and change*, ed. by M. J. ROSENBERG *et al.* New Haven (Conn.): Yale University Press.

NEWCOMB, T. M. (1953). An approach to the study of communicative acts. *Psychol. Rev.* 60, 393.

NEWCOMB T. M. (1956) The prediction of interpersonal attraction. *Amer. Psychologist* 11, 575.

OSGOOD C. E. (1960). Cognitive dynamics in the conduct of human affairs. *Publ. Opinion Quart.* 24, 341.

OSGOOD, C. E., SUCI, G. J., and P. H. TANNENBAUM, (1957). *The measurement of meaning.* Urbana (Ill.): Illinois University Press.

ROSENBERG. M. J. (1960). A structural theory of attitude dynamics. *Publ. Opinion Quart.* 24, 319.

ROSENBERG, M. J. (1965). When dissonance fails: on eliminating evaluation apprehension from attitude measurement. *J. Personality and soc. Psychol.* 1, 28.

ROSENBERG, M. J., HOVLAND, C. I., McGUIRE W. J., ABELSON, R. P., and

BREHM, J. W. (1960). *Attitude organization and change: an analysis of consistency among attitude components,* New Haven (Conn.): Yale University Press.

SHERIF, M., and HOVLAND, C. I. (1961). *Social judgment: assimilation and contrast effects in communication and attitude change.* New Haven (Conn.): Yale University Press.

SHERIF, C. W., SHERIF, M., and NEBERGALL, R. E. (1965). *Attitude and attitude change.* Philadelphia and London: W. B. Saunders Co.

11. Attitude Change and the Effects of Communication

The treatment of this area of the behavioural sciences will differ from that in preceding sections. Following BERELSON and STEINER (1964), the findings are presented in the form of short summary notes, each of which is supported by appropriate references.

The several factors involved in a communication are succinctly expressed in the question: *"who* says *what* in which *channel* to *whom* with what *effect"*. (SMITH *el al.,* 1946).

The communicator

This is not a factor about which much is known. A great deal of research has been carried out into the characteristics of leaders; to the extent that it is often the leader that communicates, these studies are relevant. But the health educator is often, at best, only a temporary leader; of more relevance to him are those studies concerned with characteristics of the communicator and how they affect acceptance of a message. Again we must stress the importance of the physician as a health educator, even when he does not wholly appreciate this inevitable outcome of his communications with his patients. This has been clearly demonstrated in cervical cytology screening programmes

(BRESLOW and HOCHSTIM, 1964; GALLUP, 1964; MARTIN, 1964; WAKEFIELD and BARIĆ, 1965; KEGELES *et al.,* 1965).

1. Although the credibility, trustworthiness, fairness or prestige of the source do not have any effect on the *learning* of factual material, such a source will result in greater attitude change than a neutral source, but this effect will wear off as time helps to dissociate the source and content. Dissociation can also occur when a highly credible source advocates a disliked attitude. Trustworthiness in the present case refers especially to the extent to which a person feels he is being manipulated by a communicator.

See: ALLYN and FESTINGER, 1961; FESTINGER and MACCOBY, 1964; HOVLAND *et al.,* 1953; HOVLAND and MANDELL, 1952; HOVLAND and WEISS, 1951; KELMAN and HOVLAND, 1953; KERRICK, 1958, 1959; MANIS, 1961 b; MERTON, 1946; MILLS and ARONSON, 1965; PASTORE and HOROWITZ, 1955; TANNENBAUM, 1956; WALSTER and FESTINGER, 1962; WEISS, 1955, 1957; WEISS and FINE, 1956. — Negative finding, ADAMS, 1960.

2. Recipients of a communication tend to agree with a well-liked speaker, and disagree with a disliked one.

See: KELMAN and EAGLEY, 1965; MILLS and ARONSON, 1965; OSGOOD and TANNENBAUM, 1955; WINTHROP, 1956, 1958.

3. Within limits of acceptance, the greater the difference between the communicator's position and that of the communicatee, the greater the change of the latter's position.

See: ARONSON et al., 1963; BERGIN, 1962; BREHM and COHEN, 1962; FESTINGER, 1957; GOLDBERG, 1954; HOVLAND and PRITZKER, 1957; SHERIF and HOVLAND, 1961; E. E. SMITH, 1961; ZIMBARDO, 1960.

The limitations referred to here include:

Personality characteristics of the recipient: VIDULICH and KAIMAN, 1961.

Assimilation — contrast effects; boomerang: BREHM and COHEN, 1962; BREHM and LIPSHER, 1959; BROCK, 1965; COHEN, 1962; DILLEHAY, 1965; HARVEY and RUTHERFORD, 1958; HELSON, 1964; HOVLAND et al., 1957; KELMAN and EAGLEY, 1965; MANIS, 1960, 1961a, 1961b. SHERIF and HOVLAND, 1961; SHERIF et al., 1965; WEISS, 1961b; WITTAKER, 1964.

Amount of coercion: BREHM and COHEN, 1962; FESTINGER and CARLSMITH, 1959.

Amount of commitment, and change possible: BREHM and COHEN, 1962.

Credibility of the communicator: doubtful credibility will lead to resistance: ARONSON et al., 1963; BERGIN, 1962; FISHER and LUBIN, 1958. HOVLAND et al., 1953; HOVLAND and WEISS, 1951. — Negative findings: FINE, 1957; KAMENETSKY and SCHMIDT, 1957.

Involvement: FREEDMAN, 1964; SHERIF et al., 1965.

The communication

The communication is concerned with what is said and how it is said. Typically, a communication intended to change an attitude employs arguments and/or positive or negative emotional appeals. LEVENTHAL (1965) has reviewed current evidence regarding the effects of fear in health messages.

(i) Type of Appeal

1. Fear-arousing appeals are effective only in so far as they are meaningful to the individual, and only if they are accompanied by a reassurance that the threat can be averted, and hence the emotional tension reduced, otherwise there is a likelihood that they will be resisted and defended against.

See: DE WOLFE and GOVERNALE, 1964; FINE, 1957; GOLDSTEIN, 1959; HOVLAND et al., 1953; JANIS and FESHBACH, 1954. JANIS and MILHOLLAND, 1954; LEVENTHAL and KAFES, 1963; LEVENTHAL and PERLOE, 1962; MALFETTI, 1962.

2. The effectiveness of fear-arousing appeals in producing acceptance of a communication decreases at higher levels of fear.

See: CUMMING and CUMMING, 1955; HAEFFNER, 1956; HOVLAND et al., 1953; JANIS and FESHBACH, 1953; JANIS and TERWILLIGER, 1962; NUNNALLY and BOBREN, 1959. WEISS and LIEBERMAN, 1959. — Negative finding: McNULTY and WALTERS, 1962.

3. The minimal fear-appeal is the most effective in producing a stable change, resistant to counter-propaganda.

See: HOVLAND et al., 1953.

4. The unfavourable effects of a strong fear-appeal occur predominantly among the chronically most anxious, the non-copers.

See: GOLDSTEIN, 1959; HOVLAND et al., 1953; JANIS and FESHBACH, 1954. — Negative finding: LEVENTHAL and PERLOE, 1962.

5. A strong fear-appeal can be more convincing than a weak one when:

a) the communication is of low interest value and the dramatic nature makes it more interesting;

b) the communication is of low relevance to the actions of the audience.

See: BERKOWITZ and COTTINGHAM, 1960.

6. Controversial material is more readily forgotten.

See: LEVINE and MURPHY, 1958. LEVINGER and CLARK, 1961. — Negative finding: FITZGERALD and AUSBEL, 1963.

(ii) Form of Communication

The forms a communication may take are many. Consideration will be given here to the superiority or otherwise of

a) primacy *versus* recency of communication,

b) climax *versus* anticlimax of communication,

c) one-sided *versus* two-sided arguments, and

d) explicit *versus* implicit conclusion-drawing.

1. There is no general law of primacy or recency in persuasion, i. e. sometimes it is the argument presented first that is most effective, and sometimes the second.

For law of primacy see: ANDERSON and BARRIOS, 1961; LUND, 1925; SPONBERG, 1946.

For law of recency see: ANDERSON, 1959; CROMWELL, 1950.

For lack of consistent findings. see: HOVLAND, 1957; HOVLAND and MANDELL, 1952.

2. The superiority of primacy or recency will depend on the individual's motivation to learn, on what and how he learns, on the temporal factors involved in measuring persuasion, on his attitude to the communicator, on his public and private commitment, and on his initial position.

See: ANDERSON and BARRIOS, 1961; HOVLAND, 1957; HOVLAND *et al.*, 1953; INSKO, 1962, 1964; MILLER and CAMPBELL, 1959.

3. Arousing needs first and then presenting relevant persuasive material is more effective than *vice versa*.

See: COHEN, 1964; HOVLAND, 1957.

4. Putting the highly desirable message before the less desirable is more effective.

See: HOVLAND, 1957; McGUIRE, 1964.

5. Familiar topics are most effective when put first; unfamiliar when last.

See: LANA, 1961; also THOMAS *et al.*, 1961.

6. Contradictory material presented by the same communicator in the same communication tends to follow a law of primacy.

See: HOVLAND, 1957.

7. What has been said in (1) and (2) above applies also to climax *versus* anticlimax, i. e. presenting the most powerful arguments last or first.

See: HOVLAND, 1957; SPONBERG, 1946.

8. Where a person disagrees with the communicator's position, or will be exposed to counter-propaganda, presenting both sides results in greater initial acceptance, or more resistance to future counter-propaganda, so long as the counter-propaganda employs different arguments from those presented in the *con* side of the communication.

See: CRANE, 1962; HOVLAND, 1957; HOVLAND *et al.*, 1949; HOVLAND *et al.*, 1953; LUMSDAINE and JANIS, 1953; McGUIRE, 1961 a; McGUIRE and PAPAGEORGIS, 1961.

9. Presenting only the arguments in support of a communication is more ef-

fective in strengthening acceptance of a communication than is presenting a refutation of opposing arguments.

See: HOVLAND et al., 1953; McGUIRE, 1961 a.

10. The effectiveness of one-sided or two-sided communications increases with the recipient's comprehension of, or familiarity with, the facts.

See: THISTLETHWAITE and KAMENETSKY, 1955.

11. Presenting a refutation of counter-arguments produces longer-lasting resistance to counter-propaganda than merely supportive arguments.

See: McGUIRE, 1962.

12. It is more effective to state the conclusions of a communication explicitly, especially in situations where the intelligence of the audience is not very high, or where the matter is complicated or unfamiliar.

See: FINE, 1957; HOVLAND et al., 1953; HOVLAND and MANDELL, 1952; THISTLETHWAITE et al., 1955.

13. Selectivity of information, especially the seeking of supportive information where belief has been shaken. See p. 54.

Channel of communication

(i) The Media of Communication

Almost as important as *what* a communicator says is *how* he says it. We have already considered, to some extent, the "how" of communication; a special aspect of this is the means of promulgation or the channel of communication by which this is done. While all the possible media of communication have been employed and evaluated and some comparative studies done of the different forms, we shall be concerned mainly with those

forms of communication that can rightly be included in the behavioural sciences.

For reviews of the media of communication the reader is recommended to consult the following: HOVLAND, 1954; McLUHAN, 1964; SCHRAMM, 1960; SCHRAMM, 1962; YOUNG et al., 1963 (A S.O.P.H.E. monograph).

Some workers in the field of communications have strongly questioned whether mass media communications can directly change or affect attitudes at all. These critics have emphasised the importance of "mediating" factors between the mass communication and the audience's reaction and have expressed a general dissatisfaction with the over-simple experimental set-up of the Yale studies. There is more to the formation and changing of attitudes than the mere presentation of a communication and the measuring of the effect that this has on a person's attitude. Having noted this criticism, we must say that it would be unfair to the Yale workers to leave the reader with the impression that they were unaware of the many factors that are at work between the communication and the audience. We deal with many of these in the course of our summary. Of special importance are the individual differences and predispositions a person brings with him to the communication situation (see p. 54 No. 3), the influence of the different way in which individuals perceive the many aspects of a communication (see p. 31 ff.) (e. g. the communicator's characteristics and position, see p. 45 ff.), and the crucial importance of the part played by groups and interpersonal communications in the transmission and the acceptance of information and new forms of behaviour. It is with this last mediating factor that many of the critics already mentioned have been concerned. (see KATZ and LAZARSFELD, 1955; KLAPPER, 1960; and ROGERS, 1962).

(ii) Group Studies

An individual exists in an environment made up of social groups to some of which he belongs. These groups may be categorized in many different ways (e. g. according to size, intimacy, role relationships, task, etc.), and studied by different means and from different points of view. We therefore find that groups are studied by different disciplines in different ways; thus the sociologist, the anthropologist, the economist, the industrial psychologist, the clinical psychologist, and the social psychologist all study groups of different kinds in different ways. Over and above this diversification of studies we also find that, for ease of management, the area of study is dissected into smaller elements; for example, conformity, cohesion, leadership, structure, function, etc.

This section will be concerned mainly with the social-psychological aspects of groups. There is a constant interaction between the individual and any number of the many groups to which he belongs. The interaction sometimes takes the form of an exchange of information and sometimes a two-way flow of forces to conform. It is for this reason that the groups to which a person belongs are of such importance in any attempt to communicate, especially when the aim is to change behaviour or attitudes.

In an effort to analyse the forces at work in the group-individual relationship, social psychologists begin by artifically creating small groups and examining the interaction processes. These artificial groups have the advantage that they can be manipulated in the laboratory; but, at the same time, their artificiality must cast doubts on the generality of their findings. Social psychologists have not been unaware of the drawbacks of using artificial groups, but it is beyond doubt that they do permit useful theoretical beginnings. Not all of the work in

this field has been carried out in the laboratory set-up; natural groups have been used, especially in industrial and psychotherapeutic situations.

The groups to which a person belongs may be classified in different ways; some are natural (e. g. family, neighbourhood) and some are artificial (e. g. the psychologists' experimental groups). From another point of view some groups are primary (e. g. the family), and some are secondary (e. g. a man's workmates). Again, from the point of view of organization, a group may be formal or informal. Common to all these differences is the fact that groups exist or are formed for different reasons, to achieve different goals, to perform different tasks, to fulfil different needs, or to provide different satisfactions for the individuals and for the groups. The origins and structure of a group will have important effects on the importance of the group, and the relative power of the group in influencing the behaviour and opinions of the individual.

The power and functioning of a group depends ultimately on the motivation that membership of the group has for the individual. Such motivation includes the attractiveness of the group members, the desirability of the goals of the group, the satisfactions provided by the group, the usefulness of the group in fulfilling the individuals' needs and goals, the ability of the group to allay anxiety, and finally the pressures from within and without the group to become and remain a member and to conform to the requirements of membership.

At any one time a person belongs to many groups of varied characteristics. He may, however, be influenced by the values or actions of a group to which he does not belong, but which he respects or to which he imagines himself to belong or to which he aspires. A useful concept to include all these aspects of group membership is that of *reference group*. (see ADAMS, 1960; GIEBER, 1960; HARDY, 1957, HOVLAND *et al.*, 1953, HYMAN, 1942, 1960; KELLEY, 1952; MERTON 1957, MERTON and KITT, 1950; NEWCOMB, 1950; SHERIF, 1948, 1953; SHERIF and SHERIF, 1964; SIEGEL and SIEGEL, 1960). A reference group may be *any* group that has power to influence a person.

It should be evident that the field and extent of influence varies with the group, but generally a reference group serves to provide the individual with factual information, with norms of behaviour as a member of the group, and with a standard of behaviour, opinion or ability against which to compare himself. (see ASCH, 1958; COHEN, 1964; DEUTSCH and GERARD, 1960; FESTINGER, 1954; HOVLAND *et al.*, 1953; KELLEY, 1952; KLEIN, 1963; SHERIF, 1958).

It is the normative function of a group that is to a large extent responsible for the conformity or uniformity of attitudes, opinions, behaviour or abilities that is characteristic of group membership. The individual need not necessarily be conscious of such group pressure. He is likely to be conscious of them when there is pressure to further the ends of the group or to provide members with a valid standard against which to compare themselves. Pressure by the group will often be unconscious when the forces arise from a person's perception of his deviance from the opinions or actions of the group.

The volume of work on conformity is already reaching unmanageable proportions; it is with this aspect that we shall begin our summary of the findings from group studies.

1. Resistance to attitude change is greater when there is greater consensus in a group which is in opposition to a particular communication, and *vice versa*

when the group agrees with a communication.

See: ASCH, 1958; BACKMAN *et al.*, 1963.

2. Pressures to conform to group standards will be greater:

a) where there is greater group cohesiveness, which fundamentally depends on the attractiveness of the group for the individual.

See: BACK, 1958; CARTWRIGHT and ZANDER, 1960, Chapter 9. FESTINGER *et al.*, 1950, also 1960; HALL, 1955; HOVLAND *et al.*, 1953; JACKSON and SALTZSTEIN, 1958; KELLEY and VOLKART, 1952; KLEIN, 1963; MUSSEN, 1950. SCHACHTER, 1960.

b) where there is greater salience of the group membership for the individual. Salience refers to "the degree to which, in a given situation, a specific group is present and prominent in a person's 'awareness'" (HOVLAND *et al* 1953, p. 155), though not necessarily consciously so.

See: CARTWRIGHT and ZANDER, 1960, Chapter 9; CHARTERS and NEWCOMB, 1958. CHEIN *et al.*, 1949; HARDY, 1957; HARTLEY and HARTLEY, 1952, HOVLAND *et al.*, 1953; KELLEY, 1955; KELLEY and WOODRUFF, 1956; LEWIN 1935, 1938.

c) the more value is placed by the group on its goals, and the more members perceive that certain actions will lead to the attainment of these goals.

See: CARTWRIGHT and ZANDER, 1960, Chapter 9; FESTINGER, 1960. SCHACHTER, 1960.

d) the more the group sees its goals to be attainable.

See: CARTWRIGHT and ZANDER, 1960, Chapter 9; RAVEN and RIETSEMA, 1960.

e) the more dependent the members are on the group to attain their own goals.

See: FESTINGER, 1960.

f) The more certain the members are that sanctions will be applied for conformity or deviance.

See: CARTWRIGHT and ZANDER, 1960, Chapter 9. FESTINGER et al., 1960; HOVLAND et al., 1953.

g) the more ambiguous the situation (social, physical, etc.)

See: COHEN, 1964; DI VESTA, 1959; FESTINGER, 1954; KELLEY and LAMB, 1957; SHERIF, 1958; THRASHER, 1954. Negative finding: SEABORNE, 1962.

h) the greater the external demand for conformity.

See: FESTINGER and THIBAUT, 1951; RADLOFF, 1961.

i) initially at least, the more a member deviates from a relevant group norm.

See: FESTINGER, 1960; SCHACHTER, 1960.

j) the less secure a person is in his position in the group — hence weaker pressure on the secure leader to conform.

See: BERKOWITZ and MACAULAY, 1961; BLAU, 1960; DITTES and KELLEY, 1956; HARVEY and CONSALVI, 1960; HOLLANDER, 1958, 1959, 1960 and 1961; HOMANS, 1961; HOVLAND et et., 1953; HUGHES, 1946; JULIAN and STEINER, 1961; RIECKEN and HOMANS, 1954.

It must be noted, though, that persons of high prestige or status in the group tend to conform highly; and popularity is positively related to conformity.

See: ARGYLE, 1957; HOVLAND et al., 1953; JOHNSTONE and KATZ, 1957; KELLEY and VOLKART, 1952; MERTON, 1949; NEWCOMB, 1950; SCHACHTER, 1960.

k) Individuals with low self-esteem are more influenced by group evaluations, and identify more readily with others.

See: STOTLAND et al., 1957; STOTLAND and HILLMER, 1962.

3) For an attitude change to be persistent, social reinforcement is necessary

from the relevant parts of one's social environment — i.e. the relevant groups.

See: FESTINGER, 1964; MACCOBY et al., 1961.

CARTWRIGHT and ZANDER (1960) limit their definition of cohesiveness to the attraction a group has for an individual. In their view, this attraction will depend on the nature and strength of the needs of the individual, and the extent to which he sees the group as able to satisfy these needs. The needs a group may satisfy may be intrinsic to the group (e. g. group membership), or extrinsic to the group, i. e. either goals towards which the group is directed or goals of the individual which he can attain via group membership. Obviously, therefore, the source of attractiveness will vary from individual to individual and will result in different forms of group behaviour.

Some groups are formed for a special purpose, to perform a specific task. Such a task-group would be one formed for the purpose of health education. The traditional form of educational groups is the lecture; how, we may ask, does this compare with the discussion-group in producing changes in attitude? The earliest investigations into this were carried out under the direction of LEWIN (LEWIN, 1943; LEWIN, 1958; RADKE and KLISURICH, 1947). These experiments were interpreted as showing that group-discussion followed by a decision was more effective than a lecture or individual instruction. COCH and FRENCH (1960), and LEVINE and BUTLER (1953) showed similar results. The conclusions were, however, open to debate, and BENNETT (1955) (also PELZ [née BENNETT] 1958) attempted to clarify the situation: she showed that the crucial factors are not group-discussion or public commitment but, rather, the act of making a decision and the degree of group consensus perceived by the individual. There has been evidence that group-discussion alone can be effective where the aim is to influence *group* goals as distinct from *individual* goals in a group setting (MITNICK and McGINNIES, 1958; PENNINGTON *et al.*, 1958). This receives further indirect support from BOND (1958) whose main findings concerned the superiority of group-discussion-plus-decision over a lecture alone in altering women's practice of breast self-examination for cancer symptoms. It is clear that further work needs to be carried out in this area to isolate the relevant factors, but certain findings can be set out:

1. Group-discussion-plus-decision is superior to a lecture or discussion alone in changing people's behaviour.

See: BAVELAS 1955. BENNET 1955. BENNETT PELZ 1958. BOND 1958. COCH and FRENCH 1960. LEVINE and BUTLER 1953. LEWIN 1943, 1958. PENNINGTON *et al* 1958. RADKE and KLISURICH 1947.

2. Group-discussion without decision is more effective than a lecture in changing people's behaviour:

See: BOND, 1958; MITNICK and Mc-GINNIES, 1958; PENNINGTON *et al.*, 1958.

Lewin's theory of forces has had a powerful influence on much of the work considered in this section. According to this theory a particular piece or level of behaviour is maintained by a balanced system of forces, some facilitating the particular behaviour and some opposing any change to new behaviour. Any change, therefore, must follow the pattern of "unfreezing" the old level, changing to the new level of behaviour, and then "freezing" the new level so as to make it permanent. When we considered "conflict" earlier on, it was noted that bringing about change by altering (reducing) the forces of resistance to change will result in less tension than by altering (i. e. increasing) the forces to perform some new

piece of behaviour. The use of group-discussion-plus-decision attempts to lower group resistance to change by individual members, and by use of the same group-power to move a person's behaviour to a new position.

See: BOND, 1958; FURUYA, 1958; KLEIN, 1963; LEWIN, 1953, 1958.

The work of KATZ and LAZARSFELD (1955) has already been mentioned. These workers, with support from many others, have postulated that communication flows in two steps from mass-media to the public *via* "opinion leaders", and have stressed the importance of *personal* communication in helping to bring about change. The adoption by doctors of the use of new drugs (COLEMAN *et al.*, 1959), and the acceptance of a cervical smear test (ROLFE, 1961), are two situations that have been examined in the light of this approach.

See: ANDERSON and MELEN, 1959; BERELSON *et al.*, 1954; COLEMAN and MARSH, 1955; COLEMAN *et al.*, 1959; KATZ, 1957; KATZ and LAZARSFELD, 1955; KLAPPER, 1960; LAZARSFELD *et al.*, 1948; MENZEL *et al.*, 1959; MENZEL and KATZ, 1955; NUNNALLY, 1961; ROLFE, 1961; WILKENING, 1956.

For the most comprehensive review of recent literature on this subject see *Diffusion of Innovations* by E. M. ROGERS (1962).

In conclusion we must emphasize again that we have only been considering a small area of group activity from a limited point of view. The aim has been to show some of the potential power of the group in influencing the individual. Finally, the group should not be thought of as a small face-to-face group; "group dynamics" aims at generalization of its results to larger non-experimental groups. The fact that much of the community-organisation programmes derive from the application of findings from the study of groups to practical problems is evidence of the usefulness of such studies.

For the best general book on group dynamics the reader is referred to CARTWRIGHT and ZANDER's book *Group Dynamics* (1960). For an excellent reference book on small group research, see HARE's *Handbook of Small Group Research* (1962) which summarises the findings (including 1385 references) without either overburdening the reader with technical detail or leaving him wondering about the meaning of the results. The same writer was co-author with STRODTBECK of a "Bibliography of Small Group Research" (1954) which included some fifteen hundred references. Of these, 584 were annotated and included in the book by HARE, BORGATTA and BALES, entitled *Small Groups: Studies in Social Interaction.* (1955).

For other books on this subject,

See: J. KLEIN, 1956; J. KLEIN, 1963; LINDZEY, 1954; Chapters by C. A. GIBB, H. H. KELLEY and J. W. THIBAULT, and H. W. RIECKEN and G. C. HOMANS; OLMSTED, 1959; THIBAUT and KELLEY, 1959.

Of special interest to health educators are the following issues of the *Health Education Monographs:*

No. 9.   1960: B. ROBERTS,
No. 10. 1961: D. B. NYSWANDER,
No. 11. 1961: I. M. ROSENSTOCK,
No. 13. 1962: C. ZANDER.

(iii) Active Participation

An important aspect of any form of education is the degree of active participation by the audience. The general conclusions can be summarized thus:

1. Active participation (by speechmaking, essay-writing, role-playing, etc.) is more effective than non-active participation in changing an attitude to bring it into line with the position taken by the communication.

See: COHEN *et al.*, 1958; CULBERTSON, 1957; FESTINGER and CARLSMITH, 1959. HOVLAND *et al.*, 1953; JANIS and KING, 1958; KELMAN, 1953; McGINNIES *et al.*, 1964; RABBIE *et al;* 1959; WEBB and CHUEH, 1965. — Negative finding: KING and JANIS, 1956.

2. The amount of change of attitude resulting from actively taking a discrepant position increases (up to a critical point) as the differences between one's initial attitude and the position one takes (in a speech, essay, etc.) increases.

See: COHEN *et al.*, 1958; FESTINGER and CARLSMITH, 1959; ROSENBERG, 1960a; ROSENBERG *et al.*, 1960.

3. Such change will be less as the strength of the forces inducing such a discrepant position increases.

See: BREHM and COHEN, 1962; COHEN *et al.*, 1958; FESTINGER and CARLSMITH, 1959; ROSENBERG, 1960a. ROSENBERG *et al.*, 1960. — Negative finding: ROSENBERG, 1965.

4. The effect of public, as opposed to private, commitment on attitude change will depend on the individual's motivation in respect to changing his attitude, the characteristics of his cognitive organization, his group-membership, and on other incentives offered by the experimenter.

See: BREHM and COHEN, 1962; COHEN *et al.*, 1959. FESTINGER, 1957; HARVEY, 1965; HOVLAND *et al.*, 1953; JANIS and GILMORE, 1965; MISCHEL, 1958; RABBIE *et al.*, 1959; RAVEN, 1959; ROSENBAUM and FRANC, 1960. ROSENBAUM and ZIMMERMAN, 1959; SMITH, 1959.

(See below for the influence of active versus passive participation in producing immunization.)

5. Public as opposed to private roleplaying produced more lasting change; such change was also affected by the

cognitive characteristics of the subjects (concreteness-abstractness).

See: HARVEY, 1965.

The recipient of the communication

The characteristics of the person receiving a communication have been investigated extensively by JANIS and HOVLAND (1959). Findings in this connection are summarized below.

1. A person will be more persuasible if he has low self-esteem.

See: ASCH, 1958; BERKOWITZ and LUNDY, 1957; CRUTCHFIELD, 1955; HOVLAND and JANIS, 1959; HOVLAND et al., 1953.
Those high in self-esteem are copers (i. e. an individual who takes an active part and tries to make the best of a situation), and those low are non-copers.

See: DABBS, 1964; HOVLAND and JANIS, 1959.

2. A pessimistic communication will produce more attitude-change among those people low in self-esteem; but more attitude-change will be produced in those with high self-esteem by optimistic communications.

See: LEVENTHAL and PERLOE, 1962. — Negative finding: DABBS, 1964.

3. Those high in self-esteem are more influenced by a communicator who is a coper, and those low in self-esteem by a communicator who is a non-coper.

See: DABBS, 1964.

4. A person who is unable to tolerate inconsistency is more likely to evaluate arguments to bring them into line with his own attitudes.

See: FESTINGER, 1957; FEATHER, 1964.

5. First-born persons are more readily influenced than other siblings.

See: BECKER and CARROLL, 1962; BEKKER et al., 1964; SCHACHTER, 1959.

6. A person will be less persuasible if he is highly aggressive.

See: HOVLAND and JANIS, 1959.

7. Females are more persuasible than males.

See: COX and BAUER, 1964; JANIS and HOVLAND, 1959; TERMAN et al., 1946.

Apart from personality characteristics there are other characteristics of a person that will affect either his selectivity regarding communications or his reception of the message.

1. People tend to expose themselves to communications with which they are likely to agree, which support their attitudes in the face of counter-communication, or which they find pleasant or interesting.

See: BAUER and BAUER, 1960; BRODBECK, 1956; CARTWRIGHT, 1949; EHRLICH et al., 1957; FESTINGER, 1957; FESTINGER, 1964; FESTINGER et al., 1958. HYMAN and SHEATSLEY, 1958; LAZARSFELD et al., 1948; MILLS et al., 1959; RILEY and RILEY, 1959; ROBINSON, 1941; ROSEN, 1961. STAR and HUGHES, 1950; G. A. STEINER, 1963; I. D. STEINER, 1962; SUCHMAN et al., 1958.

2. the above tendency is not, however, absolute; other factors will be: self-confidence (FESTINGER, 1964); accessibility of the communication (DE FLEUR and LARSEN, 1958; WAPLES, 1932).

3. The reception and acceptance of a message will be greatly influenced by the individual's motivation, predispositions or attitudes (e. g. aggressiveness, distance from proposed position, prejudice, etc.). ".... persuasive mass communication is more likely to reinforce the existing opinions of its audience than it is to change such opinions". (KLAPPER, 1960, p. 49).

See: BELBIN, 1956; COHEN, 1961; DI VESTA, 1959; FEATHER, 1963, 1964; FESTINGER, 1957; FREEDMAN, 1964;

HAVRON and COFER, 1957; HOVLAND and ROSENBERG, 1960; HYMAN and SHEATS-LEY, 1958; JANIS and MILHOLLAND, 1954; JONES and KOHLER, 1958; KANUNGO and DAS, 1960; KATZ et al., 1956, 1957; KEN-DALL and WOLF, 1949; KERRICK and McMILLAN, 1961; KLAPPER, 1960; LEVINE and MURPHY, 1958; McGINNIES et al., 1964; PEAK, 1960; PETTIGREW, 1960; SHERIF and HOVLAND, 1961; SHERIF et al., 1965; SUCHMAN et al., 1958; THOULESS, 1959; WEISS and FINE, 1955, 1956; See also earlier sections on the use of de-fence-mechanisms in the maintenance of attitudes.

4. Attitudes can be changed most easily where there is ambiguity or lack of stand-ards against which to judge them.

See: SHERIF (1958) and many of the group studies.

The effects of the communication

We have already considered many effects of communication. An important effect still to be considered is the influ-ence it has on the acceptance of a later communication that takes an opposing position. This effect is usually termed "immunization". Three of these findings were stated when considering the form of the communication, but they are repeated here for completeness.

1. Greater immunization against coun-ter-propaganda will be produced:

a) by the presentation of both pro and con arguments in those cases where the counter-propaganda employs different counter-arguments from those in the orig-inal communication.

See: HOVLAND, 1957; HOVLAND et al., 1953; LUMSDAINE and JANIS, 1953; McGUIRE, 1961a.

b) By the presentation of con argu-ments where the counter-propaganda em-ploys the same con arguments.

See: McGUIRE, 1961a.

c) by the presentation of pro argu-ments where the arguments in the coun-ter-propaganda would otherwise be dif-ferent from the original con arguments.

See: McGUIRE, 1961a.

d) by active prior refutation where the con arguments of the counter-propaganda are different from those dealt with origi-nally.

See: McGUIRE, 1961 b; McGUIRE and PAPAGEORGIS, 1961.

e) by passive prior refutation where the con arguments of the counter-propa-ganda are the same as those of the original communication.

See: McGUIRE, 1961 b; McGUIRE and PAPAGEORGIS, 1961; MANIS and BLAKE, 1963.

f) by warning the individual that his position will be open to attack.

See: ALLYN and FESTINGER, 1961; KERRICK and McMILLAN, 1961; McGUIRE and PAPAGEORGIS, 1962.

g) by providing a person with prior neutral information about the object of the emotional appeal.

See: LEWAN and STOTLAND, 1961.

2. Immunization tends to lose its im-pact with the passage of time.

See: McGUIRE, 1962. MANIS, 1965; MILLER and CAMPBELL, 1959.

3. Presenting a refutation of counter arguments produces longer-lasting re-sistance to counter-propaganda than merely supportive arguments.

See: McGUIRE, 1962.

There are several excellent works which the reader may consult. Two vol-umes in the Basic Books series can be read and understood by the layman and yet at the same time not give offence to the behavioural scientist, who will find them both useful and interesting. The first of these books is Attitude Change and Social Influence by A. R. COHEN (1964). The second book is a collection of papers by many of the foremost workers in the field of communication research, called *The Science of Human Communication: New Directions and New Findings in Communication Research*, edited by W. SCHRAMM (1963). Excellent reviews covering all the years up to 1961 are made by HOVLAND (1954), JANIS and HOVLAND (1959), and SCHRAMM (1962).

An examination of the assumptions behind, and effects of, communications in terms of the needs of the individuals to whom they are directed is made in an article by DAVISON (1959). BERELSON

(1959) paints a pessimistic picture of communication research, and is answered by SCHRAMM *et al.* (1959). BERELSON and STEINER (1964) summarize the findings in this field, as does KLAPPER in his book and reviews (1957, 1960, 1963). For a review of twenty years of public opinion research, the reader should consult the anniversary issue of the *Public Opinion Quarterly* (1957) edited by W. P. DAVISON.

Books by ABELSON (1959), BROWN (1963), and BREMBECK and HOWELL (1952) deal with the subject of persuasion.

References: Attitude change and the effects of communication

(References for the section on Group-studies are listed separately.)

ABELSON, H. I. (1959). *Persuasion*. Springer.

ADAMS, J. B. (1960). Effects of reference group and status on opinion change. *Journalism Quart.* 37, 408.

ALLYN, J., and FESTINGER L. (1961). The effectiveness of unanticipated persuasive communications. *J. abnorm. soc. Psychol.* 62, 35.

ANDERSON, N. H. (1959). Test of a model for opinion change. *J. abnorm. soc. Psychol.* 59, 371.

ANDERSON, N. H., and BARRIOS, A. A. (1961). Primacy effects in personality impression formation. *J. abnorm. soc. Psychol.* 63, 346.

ARONSON, E., TURNER, J. A., and CARLSMITH, J. M. (1963). Communicator credibility and communication discrepancy as determinants of opinion change. *J. abnorm. soc. Psychol.* 67, 31.

ASCH, S. E. (1958). Effects of group pressure upon the modification and distortion of judgments. In: *Readings in social psychology*, ed. by E. E. MACCOBY *et al.* New York: Holt, Rinehart & Winston.

BAUER, R. A., and BAUER, A. H. (1960). America mass society and mass media. *J. soc. Issues* 16, Nov. 3.

BECKER, S. W., and CARROLL, J. (1962). Ordinal position and conformity. *J. abnorm. soc. Psychol.* 65, 129.

BECKER, S. W., LERNER, M. J., and CARROL, J. (1964). Conformity as a function of birth order, payoff, and type of group pressure. *J. abnorm. soc. Psychol.* 69, 318.

BELBIN, E. (1956). The effects of propaganda on recall, recognition, and behavior. II. The conditions which determine the response to propaganda. *Brit. J. Psychol.* 47, 259.

BERELSON, B. (1959). The state of communication research. *Publ. Opinion Quart.* 23, 1.

BERELSON, B., and STEINER, G. A. (1964). *Human behavior: An inventory of scientific findings.* New York: Harcourt, Brace & World.

BERGIN, A. E. (1962). The effect of dissonant persuasive communications upon changes in a self-referring attitude. *J. Personality* 30, 423.

BERKOWITZ, L., and COTTINGHAM, D. R. (1960). The interest value and relevance of fear arousing communication. *J. abnorm. soc. Psychol.* 60, 37.

BERKOWITZ, L., and LUNDY, R. M. (1957). Personality characteristics related to susceptibility to influence by peers or authority figures. *J. Personality* **25**, 306.

BREHM, J. W., and COHEN, A. R. (1962). *Explorations in cognitive dissonance*, New York: John Wiley & Sons.

BREHM, J. W., and LIPSHER, D. (1959). Communicator — communicatee discrepancy and perceived communicator trustworthiness. *J. Personality* **27**, 352.

BREMBECK, W. L., and HOWELL, W. S. (1952). *Persuasion: a means of social control*, Englewood Cliffs, N. J.: Prentice Hall.

BRESLOW, L., and HOCHSTIM, J. R. (1964). Sociocultural aspects of cervical cytology in Alameda County, Calif. *Publ. Hlth. Rep.* **79**, 107.
Demonstrates the varying response of women at different socioeconomic levels, with least response from those most at risk. Stresses importance of physician in influencing women to undergo screening test: 90% of those tested had been recommended by their physician.

BROCK, T. C. (1965). Communicator-recipient similarity and decision change. *J. Personality and soc. Psychol.* **1**, 650.

BRODBECK, M. (1956). The role of small groups in mediating the effects of propaganda. *J. abnorm. soc. Psychol.* **52**, 166.

BROWN, J. A. C. (1963). *Techniques of persuasion.* Harmondsworth, England: Penguin.

CARTWRIGHT, D. (1949). Some principles of mass persuasion. *Hum. Relat.* **2**, 253.

COHEN, A. R. (1961). Cognitive tuning as a factor affecting impression formation. *J. Personality* **29**, 235.

COHEN, A. R. (1962). A dissonance analysis of the boomerang effect. *J. Personality* **30**, 75.

COHEN, A. R. (1964). *Attitude change and social influence*, New York: Basic Books.

COHEN, A. R., BREHM, J. W., and FLEMING, W. H. (1958). Attitude change and justification for compliance. *J. abnorm. soc. Psychol.* **56**, 276.

COX, D. F., and BAUER R. A., (1964). Self-confidence and persuasibility in women. *Publ. Opinion Quart.* **28**, 453.

CRANE, E. (1962). Immunization: with and without use of counter-arguments. *Journalism Quart.* **39**, 445.

CROMWELL, H. (1950). The relative effect on audience attitude of the first versus the second argumentative speech of a series. *Speech Monograph* **17**, 105

CRUTCHFIELD, R. S. (1955). Conformity and character. *Amer. Psychologist* **10**, 191.

CULBERTSON, F. M. (1957). Modification of an emotionally held attitude through role playing. *J. abnorm. soc. Psychol.* **54**, 230.

CUMMING, J., and CUMMING, E. (1955). Mental health education in a Canadian community. In: *Health, culture and community*, ed. by B. PAUL, New York: Russell Sage Foundation.

DABBS (jr.), J. M. (1964). Self-esteem, communicator characteristics, and attitude change. *J. abnorm. soc. Psychol.* **69**, 173.

DAVISON, W. P. (1957). Twenty years of public opinion research. *Public Opinion Quart.* **21**, *Spring.*

DAVISON, W. P. (1959). On the effects of communication. *Publ. Opinion Quart.* **23**, 343.

DeFLEUR, M., and LARSEN, O. N. (1958). *The flow of information.* New York: Harper.

DE WOLFE, A. S., and GOVERNALE, C. N. (1964). Fear and attitude change. *J. abnorm. soc. Psychol.* **69**, 119.

DILLEHAY, R. C. (1965). Judgmental processes in response to a persuasive communication. *J. Personality and soc. Psychol.* **1**, 631.

DI VESTA, F. J. (1959). Effects of confidence and motivation on susceptibility to informational social influence. *J. abnorm. soc. Psychol.* **59**, 204.

EHRLICH, D., GUTTMAN, I., SCHÖNBACH, P., and MILLS, J. (1957). Postdecision exposure to relevant information. *J. abnorm. soc. Psychol.* **54**, 98.

FEATHER, N. T. (1963). Cognitive dissonance, sensitivity, and evaluation. *J.
abnorm. soc. Psychol.* **66**, 157.

FEATHER, N. T. (1964). Acceptance and
rejection of arguments in relation to
attitude strength, critical ability, and
intolerance of inconsistency. *J. abnorm. soc. Psychol.* **69**, 127.

FESTINGER, L. (1957). *A theory of cognitive dissonance*, Evanston (Ill.): Row,
Peterson. (Stanford: Stanford University Press 1962).

FESTINGER, L. (1964). *Conflict, decision
and dissonance*, London: Tavistock.

FESTINGER, L., and CARLSMITH, J. M.
(1959). Cognitive consequences of
forced compliance. *J. abnorm. soc.
Psychol.* **58**, 203.

FESTINGER, L., and MACCOBY, N. (1964).
On resistance to persuasive communications. *J. abnorm. soc. Psychol.* **68**,
359.

FESTINGER, L., RIECKEN, H. W., and
SCHACHTER, S. (1958). When prophe-
cy fails. In: *Readings in social psychology*, ed. by E. E. MACCOBY *et al.*
New York: Holt, Rinehart & Winston. Condensed from book with the
same title and by the same authors,
Minneapolis: University of Minnesota Press, 1956.

FINE, B. J. (1957). Conclusion — draw-
ing, communicator credibility, and
anxiety as factors in opinion change.
J. abnorm. soc. Psychol. **54**, 369.

FISHER, S., and LUBIN, A. (1958). Distance as a determinant of influence in
a two-person serial interaction situation. *J. abnorm. soc. Psychol.* **56**, 230.

FITZGERALD, D., and AUSBEL, D. P.
(1963). Cognitive versus affective factors in the learning and retention of
controversial material. *J. educat. Psychol.* **54**, 73.

FREEDMAN, J. L. (1964). Involvement,
discrepancy, and change. *J. abnorm.
soc. Psychol.* **69**, 290.

Gallup Organization, Inc. (1964). *The
public's awareness and use of cancer
detection tests.* Report of a suvey
carried out for the American Cancer
Society. Princeton, N. J.: Gallup.

Demonstrates very different rates of participation in screening tests in different
sections of community: low educational
level and least well off — 28 %; better
educated and better off — 63 %. Influence
of physician stressed: 43 % of women who
had undergone cytological examination
had been influenced by their doctors. Data
taken from national probability sample.

GOLDBERG, S. C. (1954). Three situational determinants of conformity to
social norms. *J. abnorm. soc. Psychol.*
49, 325.

GOLDSTEIN, M. J. (1959). The relationship beween coping and avoiding behavior and response to fear-arousing
propaganda. *J. abnorm. soc. Psychol.*
58, 247.

HAEFFNER, D. (1956). *Some effects of
guilt-arousing and fear-arousing persuasive communications on opinion
change.* Unpublished doctoral disser-
tation: University of Rochester.

HARVEY, O. J. (1965). Some situational
and cognitive determinants of dissonance resolution. *J. Personality and
soc. Psychol.* **1**, 349.

HARVEY, O. J., and RUTHERFORD, J.
(1958). Gradual and absolute approaches to attitude change. *Sociometry* **21**, 61.

HAVRON, M. D., and COFER, C. N. (1957).
On the learning of material con-
gruent and incongruent with attitudes. *J. soc. Psychol.* **46**, 91.

HELSON, H. (1964). Current trends and
issues in adaptation-level theory
Amer. Psychologist **19**, 26.

HOVLAND, C. I. (1954). Effects of the
mass media of communication. In:
Handbook of social psychology, vol. 11,
ed. by G. LINDZEY. Cambridge (Mass.):
Addison — Wesley.

HOVLAND, C. I. (1957). *The order of presentation in persuasion*, New Haven
(Conn.): Yale University Press.

HOVLAND, C. I., HARVEY, O. J., and
SHERIF, M. (1957). Assimilation and
contrast effects in reactions to communication and attitude change. *J. abnorm. soc. Psychol.* **55**, 244.

HOVLAND, C. I., and JANIS, I. L. (Eds.)
(1959). *Personality and persuasibility.*

New Haven (Conn.): Yale University Press.

HOVLAND, C. I., JANIS, I. L., and KELLEY, H. H. (1953). *Communication and persuasion*. New Haven (Conn.): Yale University Press.

HOVLAND, C. I., LUMSDAINE, A. A., and SHEFFIELD, F. D. (1949). *Experiments on mass communication*. Princeton, (N. J.): Princeton University Press.

HOVLAND, C. I., and MANDELL, W. (1952). An experimental comparison of conclusion-drawing by the communicator and by the audience. *J. abnorm. soc. Psychol.* 47, 581.

HOVLAND, C. I., and PRITZKER, H. A. (1957). Extent of opinion change as a function of amount of change advocated. *J. abnorm. soc. Psychol.* 54, 257.

HOVLAND, C. I., and ROSENBERG, M. J. (Eds.) (1960). *Attitude organization and change*, New Haven (Conn.): Yale University Press.

HOVLAND, C. I., and WEISS, W. (1951). The influence of source credibility on communication effectiveness. *Publ. Opinion Quart.* 15, 635.

HYMAN, H. H., and SHEATSLEY, P. B. (1958). Some reasons why information campaigns fail. In: *Readings in social psychology*, ed. by E. E. MACCOBY et al., New York: Holt, Rinehart & Winston.

INSKO, C. (1962). One-sided versus two-sided communications and counter-communications. *J. abnorm. soc. Psychol.* 65, 203.

INSKO, C. (1964), Primacy versus recency in persuasion as a function of the timing of arguments and measures. *J. abnorm. soc. Psychol.* 69, 381.

JANIS, I. L., and FESHBACH, S. (1953). Effects of fear-arousing communications. *J. abnorm. soc. Psychol.* 48, 78.

JANIS. I. L., and FESHBACH, S. (1954). Personality differences associated with responsiveness to fear-arousing communications. *J. Personality* 23, 154.

JANIS, I. L., and GILMORE. J. B. (1965). The influence of incentive conditions on the success of role playing in modi-

fying attitudes. *J. Personality and soc. Psychol.* 1, 17.

JANIS, I. L., and HOVLAND, C. I. (1959). An overview of persuasibility research. In: *Personality and persuasibility*, ed. by C. I. HOVLAND and I. L. JANIS. New Haven (Conn.): Yale University Press.

JANIS, I. L., and KING, B. T. (1958). The influence of role playing on opinion change. In: *Readings in social psychology*, ed by E. E. MACCOBY et al. New York: Holt, Rinehart & Winston.

JANIS, I. L., and MILHOLLAND, H. C. (1954). The influence of threat appeals on selective learning of the content of persuasive communication. *J. Psychol.* 37, 75.

JANIS, I. L., and TERWILLIGER, R. F. (1962). An experimental study of psychological resistances to fear-arousing communications. *J. abnorm. soc. Psychol.* 65, 403.

JONES, E. E., and KOHLER, R. (1958). The effects of plausibility on the learning of controversial statements. *J. abnorm. soc. Psychol.* 57, 315.

KAMENETSKY, J., and SCHMIDT, H. (1957). Effects of personal and impersonal refutation of audience counterarguments on attitude change. *J. abnorm. soc. Psychol.* 54, 200.

KANUNGO, R., and DAS, J. P. (1960). Differential learning and forgetting as a function of the social frame of reference. *J. abnorm. soc. Psychol.* 61, 82.

KATZ, D., McCLINTOCK, C., and SARNOFF, I. (1957). The measurement of ego defense as related to attitude change. *J. Personality* 25, 465.

KATZ, D., SARNOFF, I., and McCLINTOCK, C. (1956). Ego-defense and attitude change. *Hum. Relat.* 9, 27.

KATZ, E., and LAZARSFELD, P. F. (1955). *Personal influence*. Glencoe (Ill.): Free Press.

KEGELES, S. S., KIRSCHT, J. P., HAEFNER, D. P., and ROSENSTOCK, I. M., (1965). Survey of beliefs about cancer detection and taking Papanicolaou tests. *Publ. Hlth Rep.* 80, 815.

KELMAN, H. C. (1953). Attitude change as a function of response restriction. *Hum. Relat.* 6, 185.

KELMAN, H. C., and EAGLY, A. H. (1965). Attitude toward the communicator, perception of communication content, and attitude change. *J. Personality and soc. Psychol.* 1, 63.

KELMAN, H. C., and HOVLAND, C. I. (1953). 'Reinstatement' of the communicator in delayed measurement of opinion change. *J. abnorm. soc Psychol.* 48, 327.

KENDALL, P. L., and WOLF, K. M. (1949). Deviant case analysis in the Mr. Bigot study. In: *Communications research 1948—1949*, ed. by P. F. LAZARSFELD and F. N. STANTON. New York: Harper and Row.

KERRICK, J. S. (1958). The effect of relevant and nonrelevant sources on attitude change. *J. soc. Psychol.* 47, 15.

KERRICK, J. S. (1959). New pictures, captions, and the point of resolution. *Journalism Quart.* 36, 183.

KERRICK, J. S., and McMILLAN, D. A. III (1961). The effects of instructional set on the measurement of attitude change through communications. *J. soc. Psychol.* 53, 113.

KING, B. T., and JANIS, I. L. (1956). Comparison of the effectiveness of improvised versus non-improvised role-playing in producing opinion changes. *Hum. Relat.* 9, 177.

KLAPPER, J. T. (1957). What we know about the effects of mass communication. The brink of hope. *Publ. Opinion Quart.* 21, 453.

KLAPPER, J. T. (1960). The effects of mass communication, Glencoe (Ill.): Free Press.

KLAPPER, J. T. (1963). Mass communication research: an old road resurveyed. *Publ. Opinion Quart.* 27, 515.

LANA, R. E. (1961). Familiarity and the order of presentation of persuasive communications. *J. abnorm. soc. Psychol.* 62, 573.

LAZARSFELD, P. F., BERELSON, B., and GAUDET, H. (1948). *The people's choice*, New York: Columbia University Press.

LEVENTHAL, H. (1965). Fear communications in the acceptance of preventive health practices. *Bull. N. Y. Acad. Med.* 41, 1144.

LEVENTHAL, H., and KAFES, P. N. (1963). The effectiveness of fear arousing movies in motivating preventive health measures. *N. Y. J. med.* 63, 876.

LEVENTHAL, H., and PERLOE, S. I. (1962). A relationship between self-esteem and persuasibility. *J. abnorm. soc. Psychol.* 46, 385.

LEVINE, J. M., and MURPHY, G. (1958). The learning and forgetting of controversial materials. In: *Readings in soc. psychology*, ed. by E. E. MACCOBY et al. New York: Holt, Rinehart & Winston.

LEVINGER, G., and CLARK, J. (1961). Emotional factors in the forgetting of word associations. *J. abnorm. soc. Psychol.* 62, 99.

LEWAN, P. C., and STOTLAND, E. (1961). The effects of prior information on susceptibility to an emotional appeal. *J. abnorm. soc. Psychol.* 62, 450.

LUMSDAINE, A. A., and JANIS, I. L. (1953). Resistance to 'Counterpropaganda' presentations. *Publ. Opinion Quart.* 17, 311.

LUND, F. H. (1925). The psychology of belief. *J. abnorm. soc. Psychol.* 20, 174.

McGINNIES, E., DONELSON, E., and HAAF, R. (1964). Level of initial attitude, active rehearsal, and instructional set as factors in attitude change. *J. abnorm. soc. Psychol.* 69, 437.

McGUIRE, W. J. (1961a). The effectiveness of supportive and refutational defenses in immunizing and restoring beliefs against persuasion. *Sociometry* 24, 184.

McGUIRE, W. J., (1961b). Resistance to persuasion conferred by active and passive prior refutation of the same and alternative counterarguments. *J. abnorm. soc. Psychol.* 63, 326.

McGUIRE, W. J. (1962). Persistence of the resistance to persuasion induced by various types of prior belief defenses. *J. abnorm. soc. Psychol.* **64**, 241.

McGuire, W. J. (1964). Reported in *Attitude change and social influence* by A. R. Cohen. New York: Basic Books.

McGuire, W. J., and Papageorgis, D. (1961). The relative efficacy of various types of prior belief-defense in producing immunity against persuasion. *J. abnorm. soc. Psychol.* **62**, 327.

McGuire, W., and Papageorgis, D. (1962). Effectiveness of forwarning in developing resistance to persuasion. *Publ. Opinion Quart.* **26**, 24.

McLuhan, M. (1964). *Understanding media.* London: Routledge & Kegan Paul.

McNulty, J. A., and Walters, R. H. (1962). Emotional arousal, conflict, and susceptibility to social influence. *Canad. J. Psychol.* **16**, 211.

Malfetti, J. E. (1962). Scare technique and traffic safety. *Traffic Quart.* 318.

Manis, M. (1960) The interpretation of opinion statements as a function of recipient attitude. *J. abnorm. soc. Psychol.* **60**, 340.

Manis, M. (1961a). The interpretation of opinion statements as a function of message ambiguity and recipient attitude. *J. abnorm. soc. Psychol.* **63**, 76.

Manis, M. (1961b). The interpretation of opinion statements as a function of recipient attitude and source prestige. *J. abnorm. soc. Psychol.* **63**, 82.

Manis, M. (1965). Immunization, delay, and the interpretation of persuasive messages. *J. Personality and soc. Psychol.* **1**, 541.

Manis, M., and Blake, J. B. (1963). Interpretation of persuasive messages as a function of prior immunization. *J. abnorm. soc. Psychol.* **66**, 225.

Martin, P. L. (1964). Detection of cervical cancer: a study of motivation for cytological screening. *Calif. Med.* **101**, 427.

Interwiews with 2000 women to evaluate motivating influences. Most of the 70% who had undergone cervical cytology were motivated by the advice of physicians rather than by publicity. Even among women who had been screened, knowledge of the importance of the examination and the methods involved seems generally vague.

Merton, R. K. (1946). *Mass persuasion: the social psychology of a war bond drive*, New York: Harper.

Miller, N., and Campbell, D. T. (1959). Recency and primacy in persuasion as a function of the timing of speeches and measurements. *J. abnorm. soc. Psychol.* **59**, 1.

Mills, J., and Aronson, E. (1965). Opinion change as a function of the communicator's attractiveness and desire to influence. *J. Personality and soc. Psychol.* **1**, 173.

Mills, J., Aronson, E., Robinson, H. (1959). Selectivity in exposure to information. *J. abnorm. soc. Psychol.* **59**, 250.

Mischel, W. (1958). The effect of the commitment situation on the generalization of expectancies. *J. Personality* **26**, 508.

Nunnally, J. C., and Bobren, H. M. (1959). Variables governing the willingness to receive communications on mental health. *J. Personality* **27**, 38.

Osgood, C. E., and Tannenbaum, P. H. (1955). The principle of congruity in the prediction of attitude change, *Psychol. Rev.* **62**, 42.

Pastore, N., and Horowitz, M. W. (1955). The influence of attributed motive on the acceptance of statement. *J. abnorm. soc. Psychol.* **51**, 331.

Peak, H. (1960). The effect of aroused motivation on attitudes. *J. abnorm. soc. Psychol.* **61**, 463.

Pettigrew, T. F. (1960). Social distance attitudes of South African students. *Social Forces* **38**.

Rabbie, J. M., Brehm, J. W., and Cohen, A. R. (1959). Verbalization and reactions to cognitive dissonance. *J. Personality* **27**, 407.

Raven, B. H. (1959). Social influences on opinions and the communication of related content. *J. abnorm. soc. Psychol.* **58**, 119.

RILEY (jr.), J. W., and RILEY, M. W. (1959). Mass communication and the social system. In: *Sociology today: problems and prospects*, ed. by R. K. MERTON *et al.* New York: Basic Books.

ROBINSON, W. S. (1941). Radio comes to the farmer. In: *Radio research 1941*, ed by P. F. LAZARSFELD and F. N. STANTON. New York: Duell, Sloan & Pearce.

ROGERS, E. M. (1962). *Diffusion of Innovations*. New York: Free Press of Glencoe.

ROSEN, S. (1961). Postdecision affinity for incompatible information. *J. abnorm. soc. Psychol.* 63, 188.

ROSENBAUM, M. E., and FRANC, D. E. (1960). Opinion change as a function of external commitment and amount of discrepancy from the opinion of another. *J. abnorm. soc. Psychol.* 61, 15.

ROSENBAUM, M. E., and ZIMMERMANN, I. M. (1959). The effect of external commitment on response to an attempt to change opinions. *Publ. Opinion Quart.* 23, 247.

ROSENBERG, M. J. (1960). An analysis of affective-cognitive consistency. In: *Attitude organization and change*, ed. by C. I. HOVLAND and M. J. ROSENBERG, New Haven (Conn.): Yale University Press.

ROSENBERG, M. J. (1965). When dissonance fails: on eliminating evaluation apprehension from attitude measurement. *J. Personality and soc. Psychol.* 1, 28.

SCHACHTER, S. (1959). *The psychology of affiliation*, Stanford: Stanford University Press.

SCHRAMM, W. (Ed.) (1960). *Mass communications*, Urbana (Ill): Illinois University Press.

SCHRAMM, W. (1962). Mass communication. *Ann. Rev. Psychol.* 13, 251.

SCHRAMM, W. (Ed.) (1963). *The science of human communication*, New York and London: Basic Books.

SCHRAMM, W., RIESMAN D., and BAUER, R. A. (1959). Comments on 'The state of communication research'. *Publ. Opinion Quart.* 23, 6.

SHERIF, M. (1958). Group influences upon the formation of norms and attitudes. In: *Readings in social psychology*, ed. by E. E. MACCOBY *et al.* New York: Holt, Rinehart & Winston.

SHERIF M., and HOVLAND, C. I. (1961). *Social judgment: assimilation and contrast effects in communication and attitude change* New Haven (Conn.): Yale University Press.

SHERIF, C. W., SHERIF, M., and NEBERGALL, R. E. (1965). *Attitude and attitude change.* Philadelphia and London: W. B. Saunders.

SMITH, B. L., LASSWELL, H. D., and CASEY, R. D. (1946) *Propaganda, communication and public opinion*, Princeton: Princeton University Press.

SMITH, E. E. (1959). Individual versus group goal conflict. *J. abnorm. soc. Psychol.* 58, 134.

SMITH, E. E. (1961). The power of dissonance techniques to change attitudes. *Publ. Opinion Quart.* 25, 626.

SPONBERG, H. (1946). A study of the relative effectiveness of climax and anti-climax order in an argumentative speech. *Speech Monograph* 13, 35.

STAR, S. A., and HUGHES, H. McG. (1950). Report on an educational campaign: The Cincinnati plan for the United Nations. *Amer. Sociol.* 55, 389.

STEINER, G. A. (1963). *The people look at television*, New York: Knopf.

STEINER, I. D. (1962). Receptivity to supportive versus non-supportive communications. *J. abnorm. soc. Psychol.* 65, 266.

SUCHMAN, E. A., DEAN, J. P., and WILLIAMS (jr.), R. M. (1958). *Desegregation: some propositions and research suggestions* New York: Antidefamation League of B'nai B'rith.

TANNENBAUM, P. H. (1956). Initial attitude toward source and concept as factors in attitude change through communication. *Publ. Opinion Quart.* 20, 413.

TERMAN, L. M., JOHNSON, W. D., KUZNETS, G., and McNEMAR, O. W. (1946). Psychological sex differences. In: *Manual of child psychology*, ed.

by L. CARMICHAEL, New York: John Wiley & Sons.

THISTLETHWAITE, D. L., DE HAAN, H., and KAMENETZKY, J. (1955). The effects of 'Directive' and 'Nondirective' communication procedures on attitudes. *J. abnorm. soc. Psychol.* **51.** 107.

THISTLETHWAITE, D. L., and KAMENETZKY J. (1955). Attitude change through refutation and elaboration of audience counterarguments. *J. abnorm. soc. Psychol.* **51,** 3.

THOMAS, E. J., WEBB, S., and TWEEDIE, J. (1961). Effects of familiarity with a controversial issue on acceptance of successive persuasive communications. *J. abnorm. soc. Psychol.* **63,** 656.

THOULESS, R. H. (1959). Effect of prejudice on reasoning. *Brit. J. Psychol.* **50,** 289.

VIDULICH, R. N., and KAIMAN, I. P. (1961). The effects of information source status and dogmatism upon conformity behavior. *J. abnorm. soc. Psychol.* **63,** 639.

WAKEFIELD, J. and BARIC, L. (1965). Public and professional attitudes to a screening programme for the prevention of cancer of the uterine cervix. *Brit. J. prev. soc. Med.* **19,** 151.

WALSTER, E., and FESTINGER, L. (1962). The effectiveness of 'Overheard' persuasive communications. *J. abnorm. soc. Psychol.* **65,** 395.

WAPLES, D. (1932). The relation of subject interests to actual reading. *Library Quart.* **2,** 42.

WEBB, S. C., and CHUEH J. C. (1965). The effect of role taking on the judgment of attitudes. *J. soc. Psychol.* **65,** 279.

WEISS, W. (1953). A 'Sleeper' effect in opinion change. *J. abnorm. soc. Psychol.* **48,** 173.

WEISS, W. (1957). Opinion congruence with a negative source on one issue as factor influencing agreement on another issue. *J. abnorm. soc. Psychol.* **54,** 180.

WEISS, W. (1961). Effects of an extreme anchor on scale judgments and attitude. *Psychol. Rep.* **8,** 377.

WEISS, W, and FINE, B. J. (1955). Opinion change as a function of some intrapersonal attributes of the communicatees. *J. abnorm. soc. Psychol.* **51,** 246.

WEISS, W., and FINE, B. J. (1956). The effect of induced aggressiveness on opinion change. *J. abnorm. soc. Psychol.* **52,** 109.

WEISS, W., and LIEBERMAN, B. (1959). The effects of 'Emotional' language on the induction and change of opinions. *J. soc. Psychol.* **50,** 129.

WINTHROP, H. (1956). Effect of personal qualities on one-way communication. *Psychol. Rep.* **2,** 323.

WINTHROP, H. (1958). Relation between appeal value and highbrow status of some radio and television programs. *Psychol. Rep.* **4,** 53.

WITTAKER, J. O. (1964). Cognitive dissonance and the effectiveness of persuasion. *Publ. Opinion Quart.* **28,** 547.

YOUNG, M. A. C., DiCICCO, L. M., PAUL, A. M., and SKIFF, A. W. (1963). Review of research related to health education practice. *Health Education Monographs*, Suppl. No 1.

ZIMBARDO, P. G. (1960). Involvement and communication as determinants of opinon conformity. *J. abnorm. soc. Psychol.* **60,** 86.

References: Group studies

ADAMS, J. B. (1960). Effects of reference group and status on opinion change. *Journalism Quart.* **37,** 408.

ANDERSON, B. O., and MELEN, C. O. (1959). Lazarsfeld's two-step hypothesis: Data from some Swedish surveys. *Acta Sociologica* **4,** 20.

ARGYLE, M. (1957). Social pressure in public and private situations. *J. abnorm. soc. Psychol.* **54,** 172.

ASCH, S. E. (1958). Effects of group pressure upon the modification and distortion of judgments. In: *Readings in social psychology*, ed. by E. E. MACCOBY *et al.* New York: Holt, Rinehart & Winston.

BACK, K. W. (1958). Influence through social communication. In: *Readings in social psychology*, ed. by E. E. MACCOBY *et al.* New York: Holt, Rinehart & Winston.

BACKMAN, C. W., SECORD, P. F., and PIERCE, J. R. (1963). Resistance to change in the self-concept as a function of consensus among significant others. *Sociometry* 26, 102.

BAVELAS, A., FESTINGER, L., WOODWARTH, P., and ZANDER, A. (1955). Reported *Psychology in industry* by N. R. F. MAIER. Boston: Houghton Mifflin.

BENNETT, E. B. (1955), Discussion, decision, commitment and consensus in 'Group Decision'. *Hum. Relat.* 8, 251.

BERELSON, B., LAZARSFELD, P. F., and McPHEE, W. N. (1954). *Voting: A study of opinion formation in a presidential compaign.* Chicago: Chicago University Press.

BERKOWITZ, L., and MACAULAY, J. R. (1961). Some effects of differences in status level and status stability. *Hum. Relat.* 14, 135.

BLAU, P. M. (1960). Patterns of deviation in work groups. *Sociometry* 23, 245.

BOND, B. W. (1958). A study in health education. *Internat. J. Educ.* 1, 41.

CARTWRIGHT, D., and ZANDER, A. (Eds). (1960). *Group dynamics: Research and theory.* Evanston (Ill.): Row & Peterson.

CHARTERS (jr.), W. W., and NEWCOMB, T. M. (1958). Some attitudinal effects of experimentally increased salience of a membership group. In: *Readings in social psychology*, ed. by E. E. MACCOBY *et al.* New York: Holt, Rinehart & Winston.

CHEIN, I., DEUTSCH, M., HYMAN, H., and JAHODA, M. (1949). Consistency and inconsistency in intergroup relations. *J. soc. Issues* 5, No 3.

COCH, L., and FRENCH (jr.), J. R. P. (1960). Overcoming resistance to

change. In: *Group dynamics: Research and theory,* ed. by D. CARTWRIGHT and A. ZANDER. Evanston (Ill.): Row & Peterson.

COHEN, A. R. (1964). *Attitude change and social influence,* New York and London: Basic Books.

COLEMAN, A. L., and MARSH, C. P. (1955). Differential communication among farmers in a Kentucky county. *Rural Sociol.* 20, 93.

COLEMAN, J., KATZ, E., and MENZEL, H. (In press). *Doctors and new drugs.* Glencoe (Ill.): Free Press.

COLEMAN, J., MENZEL, H., and KATZ E. (1959). Social processes in physicians' adoption of a new drug. *J. chron. Dis.* 9, 1.

DEUTSCH, M., and GERARD, H. B. (1960). A study of normative and informational social influences upon individual judgment. In: *Group Dynamics: Research and theory*, ed. by D. CARTWRIGHT and A. ZANDER. Evanston (Ill.): Row & Peterson.

DITTES, J. E., and KELLEY, H. H. (1956). Effects of different conditions of acceptance upon conformity to group norms. *J. abnorm. soc. Psychol.* 53, 100.

DIVESTA, F. J. (1959). Effects of confidence and motivation on susceptibility to informational social influence. *J. abnorm. soc. Psychol.* 59, 204.

FESTINGER, L. (1954). A theory of social comparison processes. *Hum. Relat.* 7, 117. Also in: *Small groups*, ed. by A. P. HARE *et al.* New York: Knopf (1955).

FESTINGER, L. (1960). Informal social communication. In: *Group dynamics: Research and theory*, ed. by D. CARTWRIGHT and A. ZANDER. Evanston (Ill.): Row & Peterson.

FESTINGER L., and MACCOBY, N. (1964). On resistance to persuasive communications. *J. abnorm. soc. Psychol.* 68, 359.

FESTINGER, L., SCHACHTER, S., and BACK, K. (1960). The operation of group standards. In: *Group dynamics: Research and theory.* Evanston (Ill.):

Row & Peterson. Condensed from *Social pressures in informal groups.* New York: Harper (1950).

FESTINGER, L., and THIBAUT, J. (1951). Interpersonal communication in small groups. *J. abnorm. soc. Psychol.* **46**, 92.

FURUYA, T. (1958). An experimental study of resistance to the change of attitudes. *Jap. J. Psychol.* **28**, 260.

GIBB, C. A. (1954). Leadership. In: *Handbook of social psychology*, vol. 11, ed. by G. LINDZEY. Cambridge (Mass.): Addison & Wesley.

GIEBER, W. (1960). Two communicators of the news: A study of the roles of sources and reporters. *Soc. Forces* **39**, 76.

HALL, R. L. (1955). Social influence on the aircraft commander's role. *Amer. soc. Rev.* **20**, 292.

HARDY, K. R. (1957). Determinants of conformity and attitude change. *J. abnorm. soc. Psychol.* **54**, 289.

HARE, A. P. (1962). *Handbook of small group research*, New York: Free Press of Glencoe.

HARE, A. P., BORGATTA, E. F., and BALES, R. F. (Eds.) (1955). *Small groups: Studies in social interaction.* New York: Knopf.

HARTLEY, E. L., and HARTLEY, R. E. (1952). *Fundamentals of social psychology.* New York: Knopf.

HARVEY, O. J., and Consalvi, C. (1960). Status and conformity to pressure in informal groups. *J. abnorm. and soc. Psychol.* **60**, 182.

HOLLANDER, E. P. (1958). Conformity, status, and idiosyncrasy credit. *Psychol. Rev.* **65**, 117.

HOLLANDER, E. P. (1959). Some points of reinterpretation regarding social conformity. *Sociol. Rev.* **7**, 159.

HOLLANDER, E. P. (1960). Competence and conformity in the acceptance of influence. *J. abnorm. soc. Psychol.* **61**, 365.

HOLLANDER, E. P. (1961). Some effects of perceived status on responses to innovative behavior. *J. abnorm. soc. Psychol.* **63**, 247.

HOMANS, G. C. (1961). *Social behavior: Its elementary forms.* New York: Harcourt, Brace & World.

HOVLAND, C. I., JANIS, I. L., and KELLEY, H. H. (1953). *Communication and persuasion.* New Haven: Yale University Press.

HUGHES, E. C. (1946). The knitting of racial groups in industry. *Amer. sociol. Rev.* **11**, 512.

HYMAN, H. H. (1942). The psychology of status. *Arch. Psychol.* **38**, No 269.

HYMAN, H. H. (1960). Reflections on reference groups. *Publ. Opinion Quart.* **24**, 383.

JACKSON, J. M., and SALTZSTEIN, H. D. (1958). The effect of person-group relationships on conformity processes. *J. abnorm. soc. Psychol.* **57**, 17.

JOHNSTONE, J., and KATZ, E. (1957). Youth and popular music: A study in the sociology of taste. *Amer. J. Sociol.* **62**, 563.

JULIAN, J. W., and STEINER, I. D. (1961). Perceived acceptance as a determinant of conformity behavior. *J. Soc. Psychol.* **55**, 191.

KATZ, E. (1957). The two-step flow of communication: An up-to-date report on an hypothesis. *Publ. Opinion Quart.* **21**, 61.

KATZ, E., and LAZARSFELD, P. F. (1955). *Personal influence.* Glencoe (Ill.): Free Press.

KELLEY, H. H. (1952). Two functions of reference groups. In: *Readings in social psychology*, ed. by G. E. SWANSON et al., New York: Holt.

KELLEY, H. H. (1955). Salience of membership and resistance to change of group-anchored attitudes. *Hum. Relat.* **8**, 275.

KELLEY, H. H., and LAMB, T. W. (1957). Certainty of judgment and resistance to social influence. *J. abnorm. soc. Psychol.* **55**, 137.

KELLEY, H. H., and THIBAUT, J. W. (1954). Experimental studies of group problem solving and process. In: *Handbook of social psychology*, vol. 11, ed. by G. LINDZEY. Cambridge (Mass.): Addison-Wesley.

KELLEY, H. H., and VOLKART, E. H. (1952). The resistance to change of group-anchored attitudes. *Amer. sociol. Rev.* **17**, 453.

KELLEY, H. H., and WOODRUFF, C. L. (1956). Member's reactions to apparent group approval of a counternorm communication. *J. abnorm. soc. Psychol.* **52**, 67.

KLAPPER, J. T. (1960). *The effects of mass communication.* Glencoe (Ill.): Free Press.

KLEIN, J. (1956). *The study of groups.* London: Routledge & Keegan Paul.

KLEIN, J. (1963) *Working with groups.* London: Hutchinson University Library.

LAZARSFELD, P. F., BERELSON B., and GAUDET, H. (1948). *The people's choice.* New York: Columbia University Press.

LEVINE, J., and BUTLER, J. (1953). Lecture vs. Group decision in changing behavior. In: *Group dynamics: Research and theory,* ed. by D. CARTWRIGHT and A. ZANDER. Evanston (Ill.): Row & Peterson.

LEWIN, K. (1935). Psycho-sociological problems of a minority group. *Character and Personality* **3**, 175.

LEWIN, K. (1938). The conceptual representation and the measurement of psychological forces. *Contr. psychol. Theory* **1**, No 4.

LEWIN, K. (1943). Forces behind food habits and methods of change. *Bull. nat. Res. Council* **108**, 35.

LEWIN, K. (1953). Studies in group decision. In: *Group dynamics: Research and theory,* ed. by D. CARTWRIGHT and A. ZANDER. Evanston (Ill.): Row & Peterson.

LEWIN, K. (1958). Group decision and social change. In: *Readings in social Psychology,* ed by E. E. MACCOBY. New York: Holt, Rinehart & Winston.

MACCOBY, E. E., NEWCOMB, T. M., and HARTLEY, E. L. (Eds.) (1958). *Readings in social psychology.* New York: Holt, Rinehart & Winston.

MENZEL, H., COLEMAN, J., and KATZ, E. (1959). Dimensions of being modern in medical practice. *J. chron. Dis.* **9**, 20.

MENZEL, H., and KATZ, E. (1955). Social relations and innovation in the medical profession: The epidemiology of a new Drug. *Publ. Opinion Quart.* **19**, 337.

MERTON, R. K. (1949). Patterns of influence: A study of interpersonal influence and communications behavior in a local community. In: *Communication research 1948—1949,* ed. by P. F. LAZARSFELD and F. N. STANTON. New York: Harper & Row.

MERTON, R. K. (1957). *Social theory and social structure.* Glencoe (Ill.): Free Press.

MERTON, R. K., and KITT, A. S. (1950). Contributions to the theory of reference group behavior In: *Continuities in social research,* ed. by R. K. MERTON and P. F. LAZARSFELD. Glencoe (Ill.): Free Press.

MITNICK, L. L., and McGINNIES, E. (1958). Influencing ethnocentrism in small discussion groups through a film communication. *J. abnorm. soc. Psychol.* **56**, 82.

MUSSEN, P. H. (1950). Some personality and social factors related to changes in children's attitudes toward negroes. *J. abnorm. soc. Psychol.* **45**, 423.

NEWCOMB, T. M. (1950). *Social psychology.* New York: Dryden Press.

NYSWANDER, D. B. (1961). Group dynamics. *Hlth Education Monographs* No 10.

OLMSTED, M. S. (1959). *The small group,* New York: Random House.

PELZ, E. B. (1958). Some factors in 'Group decision'. In: *Readings in social psychology,* ed. by E. E. MACCOBY et al., New York: Holt, Rinehart & Winston.

PENNINGTON, D. F. (jr), HARAVEY, F., and BASS, B. M. (1958). Some effects of decision and discussion on coalescence, change, and effectiveness. *J. appl. Psychol.* **42**, 404.

RADKE, M. J., and KLISURICH, P. (1947). Experiments in changing food habits. *J. Amer. diet. Ass.* **23**, 403.

RADLOFF, R. (1961). Opinion evaluation and affiliation. *J. abnorm. soc. Psychol.* **62**, 578.

RAVEN, B. H., and RIETSEMA, J. (1960). The effects of varied clarity of group goal and group path upon the individual and his relation to his group. *Group dynamics: Research and theory*, ed. by D. CARTWRIGHT and A. ZANDER. Evanston (Ill.): Row & Peterson.

RIECKEN, H. W., and HOMANS, G. C. (1954). Psychological aspects of social structure. In: *Handbook of social psychology*, vol. 11, ed. by G. LINDZEY. Cambridge (Mass): Addison-Wesley.

ROBERTS, B. J. (1960). Decision making: An illustration of theory building. *Hlth Education Monograph* No 9.

ROGERS, E. M. (1962). *Diffusion of innovations*, New York: Free Press of Glencoe.

ROLFE, A. (1961). *Opinion leaders: Florida cervical cancer demonstration program*. Department of Health, Education, and Welfare. (Mimeo).

ROSENSTOCK, I. M. (1961). Decision-Making by Individuals. *Hlth Education Monographs* No 11.

SCHACHTER, S. (1960). Deviation, rejection, and communication. In: *Group dynamics: Research and theory*, ed. by D. CARTWRIGHT and A. ZANDER. Evanston (Ill.): Row & Peterson.

SEABORNE, A. E. M. (1962). Group influence on the perception of ambiguous stimuli. *Brit. J. Psychol.* 53, 287.

SHERIF, M. (1948). *An outline of social psychology*, New York: Harper.

SHERIF, M. (1953). The concept of reference groups in human relations. In: *Group relations at the cross-roads*, ed. by M. SHERIF and M. O. WILSON, New York: Harper.

SHERIF, M. (1958). Group influences upon the formation of norms and attitudes.

In: *Readings in social psychology*, ed. E. E. MACCOBY *et al*. New York: Holt, Rinehart & Winston.

SHERIF, M., and SHERIF, C. W. (1964). *Reference groups: Exploration into conformity and deviation of adolescents*. New York: Harper & Row.

SIEGEL, A. E., and SIEGEL, S. (1957). Reference groups, membership groups, and attitude change. *J. abnorm. soc. Psychol.* 55, 360.

STOTLAND, E., and HILLMER, M. L. (jr) (1962). Identification, authoritarian defensiveness, and self-esteem. *J. abnorm. soc. Psychol.* 64, 334.

STOTLAND, E., THORLEY, S., THOMAS, E., COHEN, A. R., and ZANDER, A. (1957). The effects of group expectations and self-esteem upon self-evaluation. *J. abnorm. soc. Psychol.* 54, 55.

STRODTBECK, F. L., and HARE, A. P. (1954). Bibliography of small group research: from 1900 through 1953. *Sociometry* 17, 107.

THIBAUT, J. W., and KELLEY, H. H. (1959). *The social psychology of groups*. New York: John Wiley & Sons.

THRASHER, J. D. (1954). Interpersonal relations and gradations of stimulus structure as factors in judgmental variation: An experimental approach. *Sociometry* 17, 228.

WILKENING, E. A. (1956). Roles of communicatory agents in technological change in agriculture. *Soc. Forces* 34, 361.

ZANDER, A. (1962). Influencing people in the face to face setting: Research Findings and their application. *Hlth Education Monographs* No 13.

Health Education: Some Principles and Practice

12. Principles of Health Education

For a comprehensive yet manageable review of the principles of health education, as derived from behavioural studies, we can do no better than refer the reader to Section III of *Health Education Monographs*, Supplement No. 1, published by S. O. P. H. E.[1] This excellent work reviews the "Methods and Materials in Health Education (Communication)" with separate sections on: (a) fear — arousing communications; (b) pretesting and readability; (c) audio-visual methods and materials (d) group techniques, and (e) the comparative effectiveness of different methods. Perhaps even more important than the section on methods and materials is Section IV of the Monograph dealing with programme planning and evaluation. *We have not repeated references included in the S.O.P.H.E. review.*

The largely unstructured state of present-day health education should not deceive workers in the field into thinking that we talk metaphorically or euphemistically of principles of health education. Even if the principles are not as yet well-defined, there are a few that are indisputable, some that appear to be applicable to certain societies, and one that stands above all others. We refer to the fundamental importance of taking the point of view of the recipient public in all stages and aspects of health-education programming. This may sound an unnecessary injunction, but one of the most

useful principles to come out of the work of the Behavioural Studies Section of the Public Health Service of the United States' Department of Health, Education, and Welfare is that "the individual's behaviour is determined by subjective reality (defined by him) rather than by objective reality (defined by the professional expert)" (ROSENSTOCK *et al.*, 1960). In consequence, nothing can be taken for granted; careful planning is required covering each of the following points:

1. The aims and objectives educationally desirable, including both broader and narrower objectives.

2. Local beliefs. attitudes and values in the social group for whom the programme is being constructed.

3. From (2), the possible sources of motivation,

4. and the possible barriers to acceptance of the communication.

5. The resources, methods and materials available for the execution of the programme — including personnel, educational approach, media, educational aids.

6. The value and choice of the most appropriate resources, methods and materials.

7. Timing.

8. Intermediate evaluation.

9. Assessment of the results.

10. Follow-up.

Although the terms of reference of those involved in planning a health education programme are often clearly de-

---

[1] Society of Public Health Educators, Inc., 81 Hillside Road, Rye, New York, U.S.A.

fined by the instigators of the campaign, it does not always follow that the objectives are sufficiently well defined. Unless they are, proper planning and subsequent measurement of effects is impossible, and no adequate assessment of resources can be made. There are, for example, obvious differences in the demands made on medical facilities when the aim of a cancer education programme is (a) to persuade all the female population to undergo cytological examination, or (b) merely to raise the level of awareness of the population regarding possible cancer symptoms to a level which would result in earlier diagnosis of cancer. Aims can be defined in terms of actions or results in the near or more distant future; both short- and long-term aims should be clearly distinguished and defined. An example of this would be (1) the *immediate* objective of persuading a woman to go to a clinic or to her doctor for cytological examination, and (2) the *long-term* objective of persuading her of the need to have the test repeated at predetermined intervals.

The fundamental importance of a prior study of the attitudes, beliefs and values is evident. Firstly, to organize a positive programme one must know what attitudes must be changed in order that the correct ones be accepted. Secondly, local beliefs can sometimes be of assistance in producing the desired effect, e. g. the use of local religious beliefs in persuading women to be vaccinated for smallpox (BHARARA, 1963). Local beliefs can function in a curious way to impede satisfactory communication; for example, if people believe that cancer is contagious, to tell them that animals can have cancer as well as humans may sometimes result in an increase in anxiety instead of playing down the fearful aspects of cancer. Health matters do not hold a place of primary importance in all societies or

sections of society to the extent that work or family will readily be left for the sake of treatment, convalescence, etc. Local beliefs may put health matters outside the jurisdiction of human beings, or social conditions may be such that the consequences of a recommended health practice may be too serious to be permitted, e. g. going into hospital for a minor operation as a safeguard for the future when this would involve a loss of wages or even position.

The possible barriers to acceptance of a health communication are manifold. Any individually or socially held attitude or belief can militate against successful education. Such attitudes may be simply a result of ignorance of the facts, which can be easily remedied. But more often attitudes take deeper root as a result of personal experience or folklore. Several writers have emphasised the point that "communications must be consonant with the already existing constellations of attitudes, interests, needs, values, and goals of the people whose behaviour the communications are designed to change" (HYMAN and SHEATSLEY, 1958). Attitudes are held about many subjects, but those concerned with areas of life crucial to the individual will obviously be most carefully protected by both strength of belief and mental processes of defence. A person during his life develops certain fairly fixed expectations and ways of reacting in these crucial areas, and anything that threatens this personal adjustment is likely to come up against the strongest opposition; health education frequently does precisely this when it deals with matters of life and death. By raising doubts and uncertainties in a person's mind about his entire future and security, the health educator frequently creates barriers to effective communication. It is for these reasons that the most careful consideration should be given to the form the programme will take and the possible motivational effects it will have; this applies particularly to communications which directly or indirectly arouse fear. Research work in this field has shown that although fear can be a useful motivating agent, it frequently has the opposite inhibiting effect when the amount of fear is too great or where a long-term effect is desired.

Anything that is socially imposed is usually adhered to with great tenacity, but the power wielded by society will vary from one area of life to another. Society primarily concerns itself with those areas most important for its survival; among which are life, death and reproduction. Other mores and beliefs, e. g. sex, religion, are frequently maintained by means of social pressure of a more variable kind, leaving more leeway for individual interpretation, and the resulting attitudes will have to be dealt with differently in constructing health education programmes.

Other, more obvious barriers to communication are to be found in the intellectual, social, linguistic, ethnic, religious, etc., differences between the communicator and the recipient.

Successful health communications demand (a) a sound knowledge and understanding of methods and media, and (b) a thorough knowledge of the local conditions and social set-up. Much research has been carried out into the values of various forms of mass-media, educational aids, and methods of education (e. g. lecture versus discussion-groups). A knowledge of the results of this work is, however, only preliminary to a detailed review of the facilities provided by the local society in which one is working (e. g. the caste system, class system, local government set-up, clubs, etc.). Having listed the facilities available, an assessment must be made of their relative

values in helping towards the goals of the campaign. The S. O. P. H. E. review considers that "all methods and materials are useful in some program situations"; they depend for their relative effectiveness, however, on who is using them, for what purpose, and with whom. Mass media seem to have most impact in making the public aware of the problem and campaign, whereas methods involving personal contact are more effective in the crucial states of attitude changing and persuasion.

Timing the programme is crucial, both the timetable of the campaign and the period in time in which it is carried out.

Evaluation is an aspect of health education programming that is receiving more attention of late, as planners and sponsoring authorities wish to assess the results of their efforts.

Once the campagn is under way, evaluation can be usefully carried out at opportune points in its progress. Those programmes which seek some long-term on going effect cannot be finally evaluated, but in these cases, as well as in shorter campaigns, intermediate evalution is useful, if not essential. Obviously, for any meaningful evaluation, the programme objectives must be properly defined in advance.

Finally, a programme can fail due to loss of impact or motivation; for this reason it is essential to consider ways of sustaining motivation after the formal campaign is terminated. The follow-up part of a programme can take the form of reminding the public about the objectives (e. g. by posters, additional talks, etc.), or by approaching those individuals who have failed to take the recommended action.

We have already mentioned the work carried out by the Behavioral Studies Section of the Public Health Service of the United States' Department of Health,

Education and Welfare. The workers involved in this section have put forward a theoretical approach to health-behaviour which ought to be both interesting and useful, (cfr. DERRYBERRY, HOCHBAUM and ROSENSTOCK). In brief their ideas may be summarized as follows: a person's experience of a personal (or subjective) threat to his health will become conscious when he feels that he is *susceptible*, and when he feels that the illness and its consequences to him and his *own* would be *serious*. The strength of the perceived threat will depend on the relative strengths of the two factors, susceptibility and seriousness. The perception of the threat will depend initially on the presence of some stimulus or cue associated with the illness, for example a symptom of a disease, or facts about a disease which bring to a person's awareness his susceptibility to, or the danger of his contracting, a particular disease. Given such a stimulus and also the necessary degree of perceived susceptibility and seriousness, a person will take action to deal with the situation, but only on condition that the health threat is salient, that is, as long as there are not other competing motives that are felt more strongly and thus crowd out the motivation from the health threat. Although there is *theoretically* a tendency to take the action which will give the maximum protection, a person's course of action will not always be the most "rational", owing to the conflict of motives and the conflict between the pleasant and unpleasant aspects of a situation (such as going to the doctor, or having treatment in hospital). Over and above these three factors, one must also take into account the influence of social, cultural and personality factors on any form of behaviour.

Having touched on some of the general principles governing health-education,

something must be said about the special problems of cancer education. These have been discussed in detail by WAKEFIELD (1963) in *Cancer and Public Education*, on the basis of experience in England. DONALDSON, the pioneer advocate of public education about cancer in England, has also written extensively, culminating in his *The Cancer Riddle: a message of hope* (1962) which has a chapter on education.

The Australian point of view has been summarized in recent papers by RANKIN and BROWN (1964) for the State of Victoria, and by MACLAINE (1965) for the country as a whole.

The American Cancer Society has conducted a nation-wide educational programme since 1937. Since then the cures from cancer have increased from about one in five patients, to one in four in 1948, and to better than one in three at present. The Society believes its work in communications has contributed to this progress in cancer control.

The Society's educational philosophy is well reflected in *1966 Cancer Facts and Figures*, American Cancer Society, New York (particularly 'Why we say "Fight Cancer with a Checkup"...' and 'Trends in Cancer', pages 12 and 14), in *The Truth About Cancer* (1956) by Charles S. CAMERON, for many years Medical Director of the Society, particularly in the last chapter, 'The Responsibility is Yours'; in *The Climate is Hope — How They Triumphed Over Cancer* by Walter S. Ross, (1965), and in the chapter by Clifton R. READ in *The Control of Neoplasia — Education for Prevention*, (1965) which reviews the concepts, techniques, successes and failures of the campaign against uterine cancer, in which mortality has fallen in the United States by 50 per cent since 1937 when the programme began.

An Expert Committee of the World Health Organization (1964) has dealt well and yet succinctly with the many aspects of education leading to the prevention of cancer. (It should be borne in mind in this instance that the object of health education is either to prevent the onset of the disease or to prevent progression of the disease to a stage which is beyond repair). We consider that this W. H. O. report is so useful that extensive quotation from it is justified here:

Education of the public

Past cancer educational campaigns have laid stress on correction of erroneous beliefs concerning cancer and in exhorting the people to pay early attention to any sign or symptom that might lead to cancer, so that the disease could be caught at an early stage. In communities where cancer education on these lines has been vigorously applied over a long period, evidence is appearing that more cancers are being detected in the early stages.

With increasing knowledge of etiological factors and of precancerous conditions, it is time for cancer education to swing to positive preventive measures. The Committee feels that cancer education should aim at encouraging the use of the word "cancer" so that discussion of the subject can be free from secrecy and emotional embarrassment. The fact that cancer is by no means an incurable disease should be reiterated. The warnings that cancer education might create cancerophobia have proved a myth.

The problems of cancer prevention can be divided into three main classes for educational purposes, according to the persons or groups responsible for taking the preventive action:

Group I includes situations occurring in industry; education of the persons concerned [is discussed elsewhere in the report].

Group II includes situations in which there is an individual and community responsibility for coping with the risk.

Group III includes situations in which those at risk are responsible for their own protection.

In Group II problems of mixed responsibility may arise, for example in dealing with such factors as atmospheric pollution, prolonged exposure to sunlight and physico-chemical states of the soil causing radiation or nutritional hazards. Being general environmental factors they are often accepted by the population as part of life, and their danger is not recognized or resented. By their nature they may also produce conflicts of interest that may frustrate preventive action. It would be unrealistic to imagine that education alone can effect the necessary changes, but it is undoubtedly a major factor in bringing about recognition of the dangers and the will to deal with them.

Health education should therefore be planned on a long-term basis, with the aim of informing particularly the influential groups in the community of the hazards and the means of overcoming them, and of organizing collective action for their control. Apart from legislation, government action may be necessary to prepare and sustain the educational programme, and to make it easier to do the safe thing by giving subsidies and technical aid, which will underline for the population the importance the authorities attach to the measures.

Group III includes those personal habits and customs which, through their prolonged indulgence, increase the risk of cancer. The most striking recent example has been the discovery of the relationship between cigarette-smoking and lung cancer, on which extensive literature now exists. Other examples connected with chewing, drinking, sexual and marriage customs, cooking and food habits, etc., have already been dealt with [in earlier sections of the report].

The changing of customs that lead to cancer is a complex and far-reaching undertaking. Some customs, such as chewing and cigarette-smoking, are widespread and apparently satisfy important human desires.

In most countries tobacco and alcohol may also provide substantial revenue to the government and industry. History, however, does record striking changes in smoking habits. Today, the combating of deleterious customs and addictions must be looked on as a long-term process requiring an effort of research in sociology, psychology and health education at least equivalent to that expended on the clinical aspects of cancer prevention. Once the connexions have been defined and the desirable changes of habit outlined, the planning and the methods adopted for bringing about such changes will involve all strata of society and administration, backed up by personnel competent in health education and budgets envisaging long-term and wide coverage.

Promising attempts to reduce the tobacco addiction are already being made in some countries, where school health education includes information about smoking risks, and smokers' clinics use group methods to assist those who wish to give up the habit. The growing custom of serving milk, tea and soft drinks has done much to curtail the consumption of alcohol. The promotion of sex hygiene and male circumcision might contribute to the diminution of cancer of the penis and of the uterine cervix. It must be recognized that in many cases the solutions lie outside the strictly educational field.

Precancerous lesions

Signs and symptoms of precancerous lesions are recognizable in many sites, including the skin, mouth, pharynx, oesophagus, stomach, colon, rectum, female reproductive organs and breast. In some cases they can be recognized by the alert patient. Routine self-examination of the breast has proved to be a satisfactory method of detecting abnormalities early. It is sometimes argued that the association between certain "precancerous conditions" and cancer is not established. From the health education point of view the "conditions" merit professional attention on their own account, and the public should be in possession of any knowledge that may cause it to seek medical advice for them.

Health education can help to improve the prognosis by increasing the population's awareness of symptoms and by increasing their willingness to consult a doctor on what may appear to them to be trivial matters.

Teaching people to recognize symptoms is a delicate matter and most authorities are agreed that "cancer symptoms" should not be taught *per se*. The teaching should rather concentrate on symptoms that in all cases should lead the person to seek medical advice. If this is done, however, education of the medical profession will also be necessary so that the patient is treated seriously and on no account ridiculed when he does present himself because of such symptoms. The epidemiological review of precancerous conditions by mass survey methods and the more frequent declaration of symptoms by the public might also greatly improve our knowledge of etiological connexions. Routine examinations of groups at special risk is already the practice in some

countries, and health education is essential in making such examinations a success. However, there is often failure to obtain a high coverage because of poor educational planning and insufficient time for preparing the population.

Organization of health education in cancer

This has taken a variety of forms. In some countries the government has created services for cancer prevention or education. In others, powerful voluntary bodies have grown up which provide services, do research, and carry out educational work through local branches and through the meetings of other organized groups. Hospital physicians organize talks for the public. Where governmental health education departments exist they usually incorporate general information activities on cancer in their programme. The long-term nature of the work makes it essential that its organization should have continuity. The experience of short intensive programmes has not been encouraging.

The reports of WHO expert committees on cancer control[1] and on health education[2] have underlined the need for health education, and described methods whereby health education can be organized.

The International Union Against Cancer states in its constitution that one of the ways in which it believes that it can fight cancer is "by fostering, without interfering with national activities, a campaign of popular education to inform the general public of the present state of knowledge concerning cancer and of the necessity for early diagnosis".[3]

The International Union for Health Education considered cancer to be one of its major areas of interest at its 1962 Conference in Philadelphia.

Conclusions

The combination of medical action and health education, which has been so effective in combating infectious and nutritional diseases, can now be applied in the field of cancer prevention.

[1] *World Health Organisation Technical Report Series*, 1963, 251.

[2] *World Health Organisation Technical Report Series*, 1954, 89; 1958, 156; 1960, 193.

[3] International Union against Cancer (1964), *Manual*, 1963—1964, Geneva, p. 16.

In the case of occupational and community hazards, solutions often depend on changes in professional and public opinion — e. g., about social issues such as smoke abatement and about the use of diagnostic X-rays. Health education may thus be concerned with changing public opinion, promoting legislation and interpreting technical recommendations to the lay authorities and the public at large, and assisting with the organization of public action. In the case of dangerous habits, the responsibilty is with the individual and his relatives or friends and it is they who make the first diagnosis of the symptoms of precancerous lesions and who seek or avoid medical advice. Health education, as part of health services, can bring about a greater awareness and readiness to declare symptoms early. Television, radio and the press, both national and local, are powerful aids to education in this sphere and should be fully used. In the case of personal habits and customs, such as smoking and chewing, long-term health education can provide knowledge of the motivation of changes in social customs.

The educational problems of cancer prevention have not received as much attention as other aspects of cancer. There are wide gaps in our knowledge of social, psychological and educational factors that inhibit the utilization of preventive knowledge, and expenditure on research in health education concerning cancer is negligible. The organization of a long-term health education programme for cancer prevention and control is a proper sphere of interest for governments and the health agencies they control. Continuing support and the allocation and training of staff for this work are best carried out by a central ministry working through local health and medical agencies. At both central and peripheral levels, however, the voluntary cancer societies can carry much of the educational burden and should be recognized as a most valuable means of reaching the public outside the medical services. Their policies and methods should be co-ordinated with those of the government, and the research work should be shared. The

nursing professions in most countries are vitally concerned in education and their very special contribution through home visiting and group work in hospitals and the community can be utilized for cancer prevention. In order to render the work effective, both government and voluntary agencies require well-trained and experienced health education staff.

With an emotionally charged subject such as cancer, there is ample opportunity for distortion and misunderstanding, with possibly unhappy consequences for patient and programme. Only by careful pre-testing of all statements and continuing evaluation of the work by staff, can the programme's safety be controlled and its progress measured.

Education of the medical, dental, pharmaceutical and nursing professions and medical auxiliaries

As important, if not more so, is the need to ensure that physicians are cancer-conscious. The possibilities of cancer prevention have not yet sufficiently gripped the imagination of the profession. Education of the public is wasted if the physician does not seriously appreciate the importance of precancerous conditions and their immediate treatment. Dentists have admirable opportunities to deal with oral precancers. The organization of countrywide periodic refresher courses is urged.

Pharmacists, feldshers, nurses, midwives, auxiliaries, health visitors and medical workers who have close contact with patients form a valuable body for the dissemination of practical knowledge and advice on cancer, and their services can be utilized differently in different countries. They, too, should have regular opportunities to attend cancer prevention courses. It follows that in the curriculum of medical students, all aspects of cancer prevention must have a place.

A suggested programme of a course in cancer prevention is shown in [an Annex of the report].

References: Principles of health education

AITKEN-SWAN, J., and PATERSON, R. (1959). Assessment of the resuts of five years of cancer education. *Brit. med. J.* i, 708.

The assessment of five years of cancer education showed that the number of patients with breast cancer who delayed more than one month decreased. No such decrease was noted in a control area, nor did the delay for cancer of the cervix uteri decline. There was an increase in the experimental area of those with breast and cervix uteri cancer who presented themselves when the growths were of limited extent. Finally, from an interview inquiry it was found that the campaign made more impact on those with breast cancer than with cancer of the cervix uteri. One third of the patients in contact with the campaign were too afraid to act upon the advice given.

Talks were more influential than articles, but reached a smaller public.

BARIC, L., and WAKEFIELD, J. (1965). A reappraisal of cancer education. *Int. J. Hlth Educ.* **8**, 78.

After reviewing the present scientific knowledge, the authors make a clear case for the role of education in cancer prevention, and pinpoint five areas where further testing and evaluation are urgently needed.

BHARARA, S. S. (1963). Joining science and tradition. *Int. J. Hlth Educ.* **6**, 106.

BIOCCA, S. M., and JOLY, D. (1960). Fighting cancer in Argentina. *Int. J. Hlth Educ.* **3**, 174.

To succeed in the battle against cancer it is necessary to have available: (1) a qualified medical staff, able to make an accurate diagnosis; (2) a well-informed population, aware of the importance of early diagnosis; (3) a medical network that provides the essential facilities for such a diagnosis. The authors describe a campaign carried out in Argentina.

BLOKHIN, N. N. (Ed.) (1962). *Methodological Handbook of anti-cancer propaganda.* Moscow: Institute of Health Education (Russian Text).

This book contains articles on aetiology, pathogenesis, diagnosis, treatment and prophylaxis. It also deals directly with cancer education in two chapters and four appendices.

BOGOLEPOVA, L. (1962). The people's health culture. *Proceedings of the Internat. Conf. on Health and Health Education*, vol. 5, p. 520. Geneva: Int. J. Hlth Educ. (French text, English and Spanish Summaries).

BOND, B. W. (1958). A study in health education methods. *Int. J. Hlth Educ.* **1**, 41.

This study compared the effectiveness of the two methods of education, namely group-discussion plus decision and a straightforward lecture, in a health education programme concerned with breast cancer. (See page 52, col. 1 of this monograph.)

BROTHERSTON, J. (1963). Aimless benevolence . . . . a box of tricks . . . . or? *Int. J. Hlth Educ.* **6**, 158.

In a compact but pertinent article the author considers the aims and methods of health education. The objectives are both particular and general. "The real difficulty is not to find good deeds to do, but to know where, when and with what to begin". The author is in favour of tackling the "more circumscribed but necessary area [of] the quality and efficiency of the communication between the health worker and his patient or client". He condemns the authoritarian attitude of nurse and doctor; they must be made to realise the need to educate — the rest will follow. With respect to the behavioural sciences, "the need now is for a statement of applied social science carefully related to the needs of health practitioners."

Training is a cornerstone to progress, and a scientific approach to the choice of objectives is required.

BURTON, J. (1964). Three uses of health education in clinical preventive and public health practice. II. The role of education in cancer prevention. *Int. J. Hlth Educ.* **7**, 68.

This is a background paper prepared by the author for the WHO expert committee responsible for the technical report from which we have quoted extensively in the text of this chapter. The author's paper is used almost in its entirety for the sections on health education within the technical report.

CAMERON, C. S. (1956). *The truth about cancer*, New York: Prentice-Hall, Inc.,

A thoughtful round up of information about cancer and its control by the then medical director of the American Cancer Society. A vigorous expression of an aggressive philosophy of public education in cancer with emphasis on the concept that "only when everyone recognizes and accepts the importance of personal responsibility will the control of cancer become a living reality." The book has been brought up to date by the author and will be reissued by Collier Books (paperback) in 1966.

CLEMMESEN, J., and STANCKE, B. (1965). The effect of a cancer campaign in Denmark. *S. Afr. Cancer Bull.* **9**, 100.
Analysis of the long-term effects of an educational campaign for breast self-examination conducted between 1951 and 1955. The years of the campaign saw more cases, and more of them suited to treatment, than previous years. An improvement in survival was observed over the subsequent 9-year follow-up.

COSTALAT, P. (1958). Survey on Health Attitudes. *Int. J. Hlth Educ.* **1**, 207.
The inquiry proved that the health assumptions of the young Moroccan women interviewed fitted in neither with modern concepts nor with the former popular traditions. They generally combine both, with resulting incoherence and a stagnant health behaviour. Group education is the best method in these circumstances to crystallize the information spread by mass media. Simultaneous education of parents and children is needed. The author stresses the value of interviews, and the value of sometimes appealing to ideas already accepted by some nembers of the group or basing arguments on a related subject.

DERRYBERRY, M. (1958). Some Problems Faced in Educating for Health. *Int. J. Hlth Educ.* **1**, 178.
Why are people so willing to take chances with their health? There is evidence of an educational need to help people relate in a more positive way to their doctors. The "teachable moment" was immediately after the condition was diagnosed: information was sought from many sources at this point, and this, as well as misinformation, was exchanged. We must prepare people to react intelligently and healthfully when they or their relatives and friends are sick; we must help people find the information they want from a reliable source. There are many examples of the risks people take with their health, why do they do so? The author takes smoking as an example of this and considers it in terms of habit formation and society. There is need for more than a

statistical demonstration; the chance element is not referred to self, the emotional, irrational elements weigh strongly against the intellectual, rational arguments. We do not know nearly enough about the factors involved. There is a need for research into methods, and careful planning.

DERRYBERRY, M. (1960). Research: Retrospective and Perspective. *Int. J. Hlth Educ.* **3**, 164.
The primary goal of health education is to increase people's knowledge of the scientific facts about health and to stimulate them to apply the knowledge in improved health practices. Research in health education is concerned with the process by which people change their health behavior. It includes study of all the various factors in the process and the dynamics of the relationship between these factors..... The importance of knowledge, ... of social factors; .... individual factors. It is also concerned with the character of the action that is being advocated. We need to learn what educational methods work with what kinds of people to produce what kinds of actions. It is in the dynamics of these interrelationships that much intensive work is needed. We must not mistake effort for accomplishment: evaluation is essential both in pretesting and in objective evidence of the increased information and for performance of the recommended action.

DERRBERRY, M. (1960). Health education — its objectives and methods. *Hlth Education Monographs* No 8.
The author draws an analogy between health education and medicine in their diagnostic and therapeutic processes. He further considers health education as involving forces which must be analysed, a thorough consideration being given to existing "knowledge, attitudes, goals, perceptions, social status, power structure, cultural traditions and other aspects of whatever public is to be reached. Only in terms of these elements can a successful program be built".

DONALDSON, M. (1962). *The cancer riddle: a message of hope.* London: Arthur Barker.
A broad presentation of information about cancer and its treatment for the general public. It includes a discussion (Chapter 18) of the role of "cancer education among the public". Dr. DONALDSON's

ardent advocacy of public education in Britain began in the early 1930s, when his views received little or no support from professional colleagues. Such programmes as exist in Britain today stem from DO-NALDSON's pioneer work. A number of his articles are listed in other sections.

ENNES, H. (1958). Teachable Moments. *Int. J. Hlth Educ.* 1, 70.

The educational component of health activity, although continous, may vary in intensity, as, for example, in emergencies. At such moments people are potentially more amenable to education. "Our experience in 1957-58 with the influenza outbreak indicates to us that a specific health threat increases public receptivity to information, and facilitates programs of action for improving general health behavior as well as protection against the present danger."

ERDMANN. Fr. (1960). Öffentliche Krebsaufklärung als Mittel zur Prophylaxe. [Information on Cancer as a Prophylactic Means in the Fight against Cancer]. *Krebsarzt* 15, 240.

The author describes the educational aims and methods of his department for "information on cancer and advanced training in oncology".

HAMMOND, E. C. (1959). Cancer education for the public in the U.S.A. In: *Cancer*, vol. 3, ed. by R. W. RAVEN. London: Butterworth & Co. (Publ.) Ltd.

HOCHBAUM, G. M. (1959). *Some implications of theories of communication to health education practice.* Paper presented at the Seminar on Communication in Public Health Education Practice, School of Public Health and Center for Continuation Study, University of Minnesota, Minneapolis, Minnesota, June 1959 (Mimeo).

In this excellent paper the author deals with "*some* practical implications of *some* of the principles of effective communication". He begins by considering the meaning of "communication", which can be looked on as having three levels, depending on its purpose — the mere communication of information, the performance of some fairly immediate and specific action, and, thirdly, the more fundamental change of the communicant's attitudes, beliefs, and motivational patterns leading eventually to behavioural changes. Of fundamental importance is the *subjective* meaning of a message and how it fits into the already existing frame-work of a person's attitudes, interests and needs; information may be necessary in bringing about rational behaviour, but it is not usually sufficient by itself. The author continues with a very useful consideration of the timing of a communication and the best use of the "teachable moments", which are those moments created by certain circumstances (e.g. an epidemic) when there is an increased readiness to learn. Of importance for the continued effect of health communications is the sustaining of the emotional impact not only by correct timing but also by correctly spaced follow-up communications. Action should be provided while motivation is still close to the peak.

Motivation is strengthened when an action is carried out freely and for reasons that are perceived by the individual as good and acceptable, especially where such reasons are explicitly stated. These considerations also have implications for the long-term planning and integration of programmes. The author goes on to consider the role of anxiety in health communications, its uses and abuses, and its use in cancer education. An important principle in this connection is that "the anxious person looks for reasurance and not for facts". The advantages and drawbacks of mass media are critically reviewed. Finally a very useful section considers the relative merits of educating the public to accept broad principles concerning health, and programmes aimed at producing isolated actions.

HOCHBAUM, G. M. (1960a). Research relating to health education. *Hlth Education Monograph* No 8.

The author considers his topic in two parts. Firstly, the importance of discovering the attitudes, beliefs, needs, fears etc. of the individuals and social groups, prior to any attempt to influence them educationally: such factors influence what will be accepted or rejected, by whom, and under what circumstances. Having thus considered the "whys" of human behaviour, the author goes on to consider the ways and means of changing it: topics covered include mass media, group dynamics, and the theory of cognitive dissonance.

HOCHBAUM, G. M. (1960b). Modern Theories of Communication. *Children 7*, 13. Based on HOCHBAUM (1959a).

HOCHBAUM, G. M. (1960c). *Behavior in response to health threats.* Paper presented at the 1960 Annual Meeting of the Amer. Psychol. Ass. in Chicago, September 2nd. 1960. (Mimeo). See text of this chapter for summary.

HOCHBAUM, G. M. (1962). Evaluation: A diagnostic procedure. *Proceedings of the Internat. Conf. on Health and Health Education*, vol. 5, 636. Geneva: Int. J Hlth Educ.

The author summarizes the critical aspects in the evaluation of health education programmes as: "(1) Decisions on programme goals and methods, and decisions on evaluation techniques should go hand—in—hand. (2) Both the.... goals and the evaluation measures should be concerned with human behaviour. Non-observable aspects of behaviour, such as changes in knowledge and attitudes are only intermediary or substitute criteria. (3) Evaluation should be carried out as a continuous process [i. e. before, during and after the programme]. (4) Evaluation should not be considered as a measure of success, but as a diagnostic procedure that helps to identify effective and ineffective aspects of the programme". Health education objectives differ from those of a health programme: the former is concerned with the behaviour which is of help in achieving the latter (which are more concerned with medical statistics).

HOCHBAUM, G. M. (1965). Research to improve health education. *Int. J. Hlth Educ.* 8, 141.

Insufficient attention is paid to differentiating between the two kinds of research: (1) aimed at improving health education, and (2) aimed mainly at advancing knowledge. The two may differ in objectives, methodology, design, and analysis and treatment of data. Much health educational research fails because it does not adhere to principles of sound scientific research; but much fails because it adheres to them too compulsively, despite the obvious limitations imposed by field conditions. In this case compromise is necessary, but with a clear realization of how compromise will affect the interpretation of data.

HOPPER, J. M. H. (1960). The value of various forms of publicity. *Int. J. Hlth Educ.* 3, 143.

This study suppports the view that "the best way of publicising health problems is to use all the forms available, as when the four selected forms of publicity [press, bus posters, hoardings or posters at place of work, and letter to parents of tuberculin positive children] were used, attendance dropped to 88 per cent of the total attendance when the sixteen forms" as used in the 1957 campaign were employed. The results also showed that some forms of publicity attract the attention of far greater numbers of people (the first three mentioned above); prominence should be given to these in future campaigns.

HORN, D. (1956). *The attitudes of psychiatrists on the effects of cancer propaganda.* Amer. Cancer Soc. (Mimeo).

The results of a survey of 387 psychiatrists carried out in 1955 show that since 1949 (when there was also a "deliberate effort .... to de-emphasize the more fear-provoking aspects of cancer and to emphasize a "note of hope....") there has been a significant decrease in the number of psychiatrists that believe American Cancer Society literature has increased anxiety among psychiatric patients (from 35 % to 25 %). Among those believing that there has been an increase in anxiety, there has been a decrease in the number believing that such anxiety results in greater harm than good.

HYMAN, H. H., and SHEATSLEY, P. B. (1958). Some reasons why information campaigns fail. In: *Readings in social psychology*, ed. by E. E. MACCOBY *et al.* New York: Holt, Rinehart & Winton.

JAMES, W. (1964). The American Cancer Society's school education program. *J. Sch. Hlth* 34, 466.

The ACS public education director outlines concepts in a continuing programme aimed first at school administrators and teachers, to bring cancer instruction to students (down to Junior high school) "while they are in an active learning situation and before they have developed obstructive fears and misconceptions".

JOHNS, E. (1962). The Los Angeles evaluative study. *Proceedings of the In-*

ternational Conference on Health and Health Education, vol. 5, 514. Geneva: Int. J. Hlth Educ.

This study was designed to evaluate the effectiveness of school health education. The effectiveness of health education was judged by means of an appraisal of the programme activities and the health behaviour of pupils in terms of knowledge, attitudes and practices.

KATSUNUMA, H. (1958). Before planning: a survey. *Int. J. Hlth Educ.* 1, 151.

To help determine the best health education approach in a rural community, a survey on family attitudes regarding health problems was recently undertaken in a district near Tokyo.

KING, S. H. (1958). What we can learn from the behavioural sciences. *Int. J. Hlth Educ.* 1, 194.

The author stresses the importance of familiarity with the major concepts of the behavioural sciences, and their integration across the biological, psychological and social-cultural levels. "They [public health workers] also need to be introduced to the findings of research projects that are pertinent to an understanding of disease and of social factors that inhibit or facilitate health programmes." The major concepts considered are: social perception or definition of the situation, homeostasis or a striving towards a balance, beliefs and attitudes, and political structures and communication lines.

KNUTSON, A. L. (1952a). Evaluating health education. *Publ. Hlth Rep.* 67, 73.

In the evaluation of any health education programme one should consider the following points: adequate preliminary investigation should be made to ascertain needs and behaviour; goals must be specified, but evaluated in relation to the overall aims; concrete evidence that an objective has been achieved is the only realistic criterion for measuring effectiveness; methods of evaluation must be chosen in terms of the specific goals; a baseline of zero cannot be presumed; evaluative measurements are nearly always indirect measures; long-term needs should be borne in mind apart from the immediate goals.

KNUTSON, A. L. (1952b). Pretesting: A positive approach to evaluation. *Publ. Hlth Rep.* 67, 699.

A critical review should be made prior to pretesting a programme so that the needs, objectives, methods, and subject matter are clearly defined, accurate and likely to be most successful. The pretest should be planned in terms of certain specific conditions that need to be satisfied in order to achieve programme goals; the programme will then be more likely to succeed. The conditions to be satisfied include: amount of public exposure, attention and interest, motivation, pattern of behaviour, comprehension, understanding of purpose, learning and retention.

KNUTSON, A. L., SHIMBERG, B., HARRIS, J. S., and DERRYBERRY, M. (1952). Pretesting and evaluating health education. *Publ. Hlth Monograph* No 8. Washington, D. C.: United States Public Health Service Publication No 212.

KOCH, F., and STAKEMANN, G. (1964). A population screening for carcinoma of the uterus with the irrigation smear technique. *Dan. med. Bull.* 11, 209.

A remarkable project in the borough of Frederiksberg, Copenhagen, appears to demonstrate the acceptability of self-obtained smears (by pipette) without major educational effort. Of 11,192 selected women, 82.2 % used and returned the pipettes. Propaganda limited to one 3-minute interview on T. V. and a few items in newspapers. The authors suggest this success is due to the fact that women can undertake the procedure in the privacy of their homes, and without the inconvenience or embarrassment of making an appointment for examination.

LA POINTE, J. L., WITTKOWER, E. D., and LOUGHEED, M. N. (1959). Psychiatric evaluation of the effect of cancer education on the lay public. *Cancer* (Philad.) 12, 1200.

The authors believe that cancer education and many other forms of health education have relatively little effect considering the amounts of time, money and skill spent on them. There is a reliance on the mass media, merely presenting material to large groups of individuals regardless of their receptivity. A more personal approach through discussion groups and the like may produce a lessening of resistances and thus reduce the blocking reactions. Once the general public has allowed itself to be exposed to education, greater resistances might be overcome if other factors, such as the different needs of the population, or which person is more liable to be heard and understood in specific groups, were known. "The real problem is not whether enough information is put across to the general public, but how and how successfully the information is communicated. There is little doubt in our minds, for instance, that propaganda based on curability through early treatment is more likely to be successful than is propaganda based on fear."

LIFSON, S. S. (1958). Do they understand what they read? *Int. J. Hlth Educ.* 1, 100.

Giving literature to patients in hospitals is not enough. We must find out if they understand what they read. An interesting survey was carried out in this connection by the U.S. Tuberculosis Association, making use of reading tests. It proved two things: the need for hospital personnel to be aware of the level of vocabulary comprehension of their patients; and, secondly, that we should not rely mainly on the printed word for our educational effort.

McCORMICK, G. (1964). Programme planning — An organized approach. *Int. J. Hlth Educ. 7, 91.*

The author discusses how he used the W.H.O. guide to programme — planning when he was co-ordinator of a community nursing-home demonstration programme. The W.H.O. guide enumerated the following five steps: (1) collecting information essential for planning; (2) establishment of objectives; (3) assessing the barriers to health education and how they may be overcome; (4) appraising apparent and potential resources (organisations, personnel, materials and funds); (5) developing the detailed educational plan of operations (including a definite mechanism for continuous evaluation).

MACLAINE, A. G. (1965). Lay education in cancer control. *Med. J. Aust.* 2, 171.

A succinct review of experience elsewhere and discussion of possible applications to the situation in Australia. This article is not written from a limited parochial point of view, and its interest is therefore not confined to the country of origin.

McNICKLE, d'A., and PFROMMER, V. G. (1959). It takes two to communicate. *Int. J. Hlth Educ.* 2, 136.

NIX, M. E. (1961). Health education and human motivation. *Int. J. Hlth Educ.* 4, 192.

Although the importance of health and illness has global significance, attitudes regarding these will vary according to the cultural ideals of a community. Therefore, although the problem of the control of tuberculosis is universal, it can be solved by giving careful consideration to the fixed customs of the group. The author considers the different types of atmosphere of a group associated with the types of leadership, and the consequences for human motivation and behaviour. If the leader is authoritarian or laissez—faire the positive results, if any, are unlikely to be permanent. Ideally the relationship should be one of educated self-determination, in which a person follows a responsible leader with understanding and the realization that the programme will benefit him and those around him.

OSBORN, G. R., and LEYSHON, V. N. (1966). Domiciliary testing of cervical smears by home nurses. *Lancet* 1, 256.

Public health nurses in Derby were used in a cervical cytology programme (a) to identify the high-risk women (multiparous, low on socio-economic scale) in their care; (b) to persuade them to have a smear taken; (c) to take smears (after careful training) in the home. The value of this highly personal form of selective health education was shown by results. Moreover, a positive smear rate of 26.5 per 1000 was found in this group, almost four times greater than the rate recorded for the general population at clinics in the same town.

PATERSON, R., and AITKEN-SWAN, J. (1954). Public opinion on cancer: A survey among women in the Manchester area. *Lancet* ii, 857.

A report of the first survey carried out at the beginning of the experimental cancer education programme by the Manchester Committee on Cancer. (See Chapter I of this Monograph).

PATERSON, R., and AITKEN-SWAN, J. (1958). Public opinion on cancer: Changes following five years of cancer education. *Lancet* ii. 791.

This is a repeat survey of the one carried out in 1953 (Paterson and Aitken-Swan 1954) and showed a good general improvement in attitudes to cancer. (See Chapter I of this Monograph).

PATERSON, R., Brown, C. M., and WAKE-FIELD, J. (1954). An experiment in cancer education. *Brit. med. J.* ii, 1219.
This is an early article describing the cancer education programme of the Manchester Committee on Cancer.

PHILLIPS, A. J. (1955). Public opinion on cancer in Canada. *Canad. med. Ass. J.* 73, 639. (See Chapter I of this report).

PHILLIPS, A. J., and TAYLOR, R. M. (1961). Public opinion on cancer in Canada; a second survey. *Canad. med. Ass. J.* 84, 142.
This is a report on a repeat of the 1955 survey (Phillips 1955), and shows an improvement in public opinion concerning cancer after a carefully planned educational campaign. (See Chapter I of this report).

POPMA, A. M. (1962). Public education and cancer control. *Acta Uni. int. Cancr.* 18, 723.
The author deals with the history of public cancer education both in the United States and Great Britain. Fear of cancer needs to be eradicated by education organised by the medical profession. Much evidence is cited to show the value of early diagnosis of cancer of all sites, especially asymptomatic cancer.
Cancerophobia, the most common objection to education, is not a true problem. It should be guided by education into a salutary fear of undue delay in seeking adequate treatment.

PRICE-WILLIAMS, D. R. (1962). New attitudes emerge from the old. *Proceedings of the International Conference on Health and Health Education,* vol. 5, 554. Geneva: International Journal of Health Education.
The author emphasizes the importance of taking into account the background of ideas and practices in health education. New ideas must be seen in relation to the old ones that they are disrupting or replacing. The author illustrates his points

with examples from a tribe he studied in Nigeria.

RANKIN, D. W., and BROWN, A. J. (1964). Cancer education in Victoria. *Med. J. Aust.* 1, 357.
A description of five years of intensive cancer education of the public by the Anti-cancer Council of Australia, its organization objectives, methods and evaluation.

RAVEN, R. W., (1953). Cancer and the community. *Brit. med. J.* ii, 850.
Among other topics, he discusses a cancer education programme. Telling the public the symptons is not enough, they must also be told how to act in certain circumstances, and what can be done to help them. This must be done wisely and in stages throughout the country.

READ, C. R. (1965). The control of neoplasia — education for prevention. In: *The social responsibility of gynecology and obstetrics.* Baltimore: Johns Hopkins Press.
The American Cancer Society's vice president for public education and information reviews his and the Society's experience in many years of education against cancer of the uterus. He emphasizes the need for physician leadership, the importance of terminology acceptable to the media and meaningful to the public, the need to use both media and person-to-person approaches through informal networks of communication, (churches, unions, women's clubs, neighbourhoods, etc.), the educational stress on "hope, on the peace of mind the Pap test can give". Many millions in America have learned a new health habit, but there has been too little success with low-income groups and women over the age of 65. The diffusion process in health education is slow.

ROBERTS, B. J. (1965). A framework for consideration of forces in achieving earliness of treatment. *Hlth Education Monographs* No 19.
A stimulating analysis of the motivational and other forces involved in achieving early detection and treatment, particularly of breast cancer, by health educational methods. Invaluable because it offers for the first time a holistic view of the decision-making forces that lead to action, rather than the usual fragmentary examination of some aspects of the problem.

ROBERTS, B. J. (1962). Concepts and methods of evaluation in health education. *Int. J. Hlth Educ.* **5**, 52.

In this article the author attempts to clarify the concepts surrounding evaluation in health education, and considers the problems of measurement involved in such evaluation.

ROSENSTOCK, I. M., HOCHBAUM, G. M., and KEGELES, S. S. (1960). *Determinants of health behavior.* Golden Anniversary White House Conference on Children and Youth. See the text of this chapter for a summary.

ROSENSTOCK, I. M. (1960). Gaps and potentials in health education research. *Hlth Education Monographs* No 8.

The author considers that applied research is needed to "develop simple, economical and valid methods for diagnosing health education problems; [and also] . . . to develop valid methods for educating individuals and groups in a real life health setting". Further "basic research is needed to increase our growing knowledge of why people do what they do". Finally, much more programme evaluation is required to help in improving programmes.

ROSENSTOCK, I. M. (1961). Decision-making by individuals. *Hlth Education Monographs* No 11. See the text of this chapter for summary.

ROSENSTOCK, I. M. (1962). Many opinions. . . Few Hard Facts. *Proceedings of the International Conference on Health and Health Education,* vol. 5, 565. Geneva: Int. J. Hlth Educ.

The author is of the opinion that "what we still do not know . . . . is how best to *diagnose* and *use* existing motivational states and existing social structures to change behaviour".

ROSENSTOCK, I. M. (1963). Public response to cancer screening and detection programs. *J. chron. Dis.* **16**, 407.

In the second part of the paper, Rosenstock attempts to apply the behavioural model already developed (see text of chapter) to cancer detection.
The research that is required should be directed at the groups shown to be in need of it by a consideration of their health behaviour status — e. g. the undermotivated. The author concludes with recommendations for (a) a fact-finding phase; and (b) an action phase.

ROSS, W. S. (1965). *The climate is hope — How they triumphed over cancer,* New York: Prentice-Hall, Inc.

The book reports the personal attitudes to cancer of physicians, their patients, most of whom have been cured, and researchers. Sixteen rambling chapters — largely taped interviews — reflect the fears and guilt of some patients, the courage of others. Physicians speak candidly of their limitations as well as their successes: one is deeply interested in problems of stress and cancer, another in the value of a cancer detection examination, a third in the philosophy of radical operations, a fourth in the unbearable family tensions that often develop when a child has cancer. "Cancer is a highly complex group of diseases, each with its own course and prognosis . . . Hence the reactions and the judgements of both patients and therapists often vary greatly and may be controversial."

SANDMAN, I. (1962). Parent education in the U. S. A: Some impressions on methods. *Int. J. Hlth Educ.* **5**, 34.

The author examined whether group discussions would produce better results than the traditional courses in health education of expectant mothers. The answer appears to be in the affirmative. Although factual information is important, an understanding of one's feelings is also important and both are achieved in discussions.

SEPPILLI, A. (1962). A community survey — First step towards a film. *Proceedings of the International Conference on Health and Health Education,* vol. 5, 527. Geneva: Int. J. Hlth Education. (French text, English and Spanish Summaries).

SPILLIUS, J. (1962). The impact of social structure. *Proceedings of the International Conference on Health and Health Education,* vol. 5, 560. Geneva: Int. J. Hlth Educ.

The author suggests "(1) that the health educator may have to redefine the kind of system he is dealing with; (2) that a health education programme may constitute a direct attack on some of the individuals in the community, especially those who hold some kind of medical lore; (3) that it is necessary to study the customary ways of imparting information, recognizing that there may be an informal [social] structure, such as a network of kin which is just as potent as the formal structure in imparting information and shaping opinion; (4) that it is necessary to make a distinction between decision-making and choices..., (5) that cultures change, customs change, and in some societies at a more rapid rate than in others.... it should [therefore] be possible to change ideas on health and disease if we analyse the social patterns, see who is responsible for health practices, and whether or not the community's ideas are really as irrational as they appear. In attempting to promote change, we should obviously use the existing social structure as much as possible". Society should not be looked at in terms of social structure alone; health education programmes affect the social, economic and technological structures, and these three aspects must be included in the planning and execution of the programme. The physical and economic burden placed on the people of a developing country must be borne in mind in any health education programme.

STEUART, G. (1965). The physician and health education. *Brit. med. J.* ii, 590.

The author considers that the passive role of the patient is not conducive to good health education *via* the doctor, and recommends that the relationship be changed to a more patient-oriented one, in which the latter plays an active part. Steuart deals with the reasons why a patient should be educated, possible objections to his proposals, and the part played in all this by basic medical education of the doctor.

STEUART, G. (1959). The importance of programme planning. *Int. J. Hlth Educ.* 2, 94.

Systematic and intelligent planning are essential for successful health education. (See text of this chapter). Illustrations are taken from a programme concerning ante-natal and maternity care in a South African Indian community.

STEUART, G. (1962). A slender store of studies... *Proceedings of the International Conference on Health and Health Education*, vol. 5, 608. Geneva: Int. J. Hlth Educ.

In this very instructive article the author reviews the studies of the educational content of health education programmes. Such studies are concerned with evaluation of the effectivenness of programmes, the existence and extent of the problem in the community or group, the establishment of criteria or baselines against which to measure and compare results, the comparative effectiveness of methods and the use of methods appropriate to the population and problem. More such studies are needed, and the help of the pure scientist must be used wherever possible. This article includes a bibliography of nearly fifty articles.

SUCHMAN, E. (1962). More scientific rigour is needed. *Proceedings of the International Conference on Health and Health Education*, vol. 5, 533. Geneva: Int. J. Hlth Educ.

A great deal more thought might be given to the problem of classification of research findings, but this would involve the clarification of the basic dimensions underlying its fundamental concepts. Only by attempting to relate findings to such concepts will the results of applied research be of use outside the limited experimental situation. The research design of most health education studies is weak, owing to lack of underlying theory; they also lack scientific rigour. There are many possible criteria for the evaluation of an educational programme — in terms of effort, performance, adequacy, efficiency —, effort is the most common. Health education must develop its objectives more specifically according to different degrees of immediacy; this will necessitate an examination of the basic assumptions concerning the goals involved.

SUSTAITA SEEBER, A. de (1963). Changing attitudes to cancer. *Int. J. Hlth Educ.*, 6, 88.

The results of a cancer education campaign in Argentina showed that attitudes to cancer have improved: information was sought and accepted more frequently, there was less delay by patients, conversations about cancer were considered more natural, and the educational approach is much more optimistic in outlook.

TENTORI, F. V. (1962). Their needs and knowledge. *Int. J. Hlth Educ.*, **5**, 10.

With ample illustration the author emphasizes the importance of preliminary research and evaluation in the careful planning of a programme. The research should include an examination of the characteristics and attitudes of the community.

TENTORI, F. V. (1963). Audio-visual materials: an experiment in pretesting. *Int. J. Hlth Educ.*, **6**, 180.

This article sums up ... the results of a study carried out by the author in Mexico. The purpose was to pretest audio-visual materials being planned to support a public health programme....
The results emphasize the value of such tests and pinpoint some important principles.

WAKEFIELD, J. (1959). The case for cancer education. *Monthly Bulletin of the Ministry of Health and the Public Health Laboratory Service* **18**, 146.

The arguments for and against public education about cancer are presented and examined in the light of available evidence. The evidence shows that a carefully conceived and tactfully executed programme of education does not have undesirable effects, and that it can favourably influence public attitudes to cancer.

WAKEFIELD, J. (1963). *Cancer and public education.* London: Pitman Med. Publ. Co. Ltd; Springfield (Ill.): Ch. C. Thomas.

This volume summarizes many years in the field of cancer education in England. Probably the only work devoted solely to cancer education. Topics covered in the different chapters include: the principles and practice of cancer education — the problem, delay in seeking treatment, the content of a programme, informing the public by mass-media and person-to-person methods, cancer education in schools and the smoking problem —, and the organization of public education schemes. The appendices contain notes for lecturers, a reprint of the Paterson and Aitken-Swan (1954) survey, notes on the use of visual aids, and a list of educational materials and sources.

WAKEFIELD, J. (1966). The role of public education in cancer detection. In:

Chap.-VI., UICC Monograph Ser., vol. 4. Berlin-Heidelberg-New York: Springer 1966.

The author emphasises that detection programmes must be accompanied by public education. The objectives of such education must be "to persuade people to seek prompt medical advice when certain warning signs appear; and to persuade them particularly those in high-risk groups, to take part in screening programmes"; emphasis on the hopeful and reassuring aspects of cancer and cancer detection tests is important. The author deals with the functions of the physician, other medical staff, and mass-media in education for detection of cancer. Crucial, however, in any such education is the state of the attitudes, beliefs and health practices in the community or group being educated. Wakefield draws attention to the need for examining the qualities of detection tests that attract or repel an individual, and cause him to accept or reject the test. The article is supported with evidence from a number of relevant studies.

WAKEFIELD, J., and DAVISON, R. L. (1958). An answer to some criticisms of cancer education: A survey among general practitioners. *Brit. med. J.* i, 96.

This is a report of a survey carried out after five years of public education. It was designed to test the validity of the criticisms "that cancer education would create cancerophobia among the public and add unnecessarily to the work of the general practitioners". Such criticisms were shown to be invalid for the kind of educational programme used.

WHO (1963). Cancer control. *Wld Hlth Org. Tech. Rep. Ser.* No **251**.

This report contains a short section on education of the public, in which a few notes are made on the most important points of such education: necessity, form and operation of cancer education.

WHO (1964). Prevention of cancer. *Wld Hlth Org. Rep. Ser.* No **276**.

This report contains an excellent section on public education, which we have quoted extensively in the text of the chapter.

YOUNG, M. A. C., DiCicco, L. M., PAUL, A. M., and SKIFF, A. W. (1963). *Review of research related to health education practice. Hlth Education*

Monographs, Suppl. No 1. New York: Society of Public Educators, Inc.

ZABOLOTSKAIA, L. (1965). The integration of health education in preventive and curative medicine in the U.S.S.R. *Int. J. Hlth Educ.,* 8, 41.

Prophylactic examination of healthy people is carried out in various selected categories of the population. A widespread educational effort precedes such examination programmes to ensure maximum participation. Follow-up of the chronic sick revealed by examination is tackled systematically, with health education playing a major role.

Ministry of Health, London (1964). *Health education.* Report of a Joint Committee of the Central and Scottish Health Services Councils. London: Her Majesty's Stationery Office.

This excellent report deals with the aims and achievements of health education. The need for evaluation is stressed and the future organization of health education in Britain is considered. Finally, the report deals with the techniques of health educators, the part played by general practitioners, and health education in schools. An appendix on health education

in the United States is included. There are several lengthy comments on health education about cancer.

Many methods useful for evaluation in health education. *Int. J. Hlth Educ.* 5, 93. [Editorial annotation].

Lists ten of a variety of methods that have been used to check changes in knowledge, attitudes and behaviour of students relating to health.

Health Education: a selected bibliography prepared by the World Health Organization. (1956). *Educational Studies and Documents.* No XIX. Paris: UNESCO.

174 entries on (1) General background; (2) Health education; (3) Methods and techniques; (4) Training; (5) Evaluation (6) Periodicals.

Health Education (1962), *Education Abstracts,* vol. XVI, No 1, compiled by *Winifred Warden.* Paris: UNESCO.

An annotated bibliography of 398 entries on (1) Philosophy and background; (2) school health; (3) Programme planning; (4) Problems in special fields (including smoking); (5) Books for children; (6) Periodicals of interest.

13. Aims and Methods of Current Cancer Education Programmes in Various Countries

To describe in detail cancer education programmes throughout the world would be impossible, and pointless in the present context. The information in this chapter is therefore intended as no more than an indication of how theory is being put into practice in a few countries. It is extracted from detailed working papers[1] regarding their own regions prepared by members of the Committee on Public Education of the International Union against Cancer.

Several themes run consistently through all current cancer education programmes — to disseminate *reliable* information about cancer, to eliminate irrational fears of the disease, and to promote diagnosis at the earliest possible stage, whether by seeking advice promptly for signs and symptoms recognizable by the patient or, more recently, by making use of measures of detection and prevention available. Not unexpectedly, there are differences in the way in which different coutries seek to achieve these aims, but we see these as variations in interpretation, perhaps allied to differences in national customs, systems of communication and mores, rather than as differences of principle.

[1] The collected papers, *Public Education: Cancer Education Programmes in Various Countries,* are available from U. I. C. C. Geneva Office, 3 rue du Conseil-Général, Geneva, Switzerland, in the form of a Technical Report.

What follows is therefore a brief sketch of how the problem is tackled in various countries, and not an attempt to compare and synthesize the differences which exist.

Australia

The Australian Cancer Society, a federation of state anti-cancer organizations, was formed in 1961. The objectives of its Public Education Committee include fostering and co-ordinating public education activities throughout Australia; the preparation of a blue-print for a public education campaign which could be implemented by any organization which so desired; the establishment of a means of examination of methods of communication to determine the effect of public education on cancer; the provision of a means of pre-testing public reactions to new educational material before its release for general exhibition; dissemination of information and educational material on cancer from all Australian States and overseas countries.

The main emphasis in cancer education has been placed on those methods offering a more personal type of approach. Most important of these is the illustrated talk to an existing community group, in which simple but accurate information can be given that will enable the layman to recognize certain symptoms as possible signs of cancer, increase his understanding of the disease, and counter some of the prevailing fallacies and misconceptions. Full use is made of audio-visual aids — films, filmstrips, slides and tape recordings — to aid audience comprehension of the lectures.

Although the percentage of the total population reached in this way will not be large, regular work with these organizations can create what WAKEFIELD terms "a nucleus of well-informed people in the community" whose influence may spread far beyond the confines of their immediate circle of relative and friends.

While it is recognized that an education effort concentrated on the mass media is less likely to bring about any significant and lasting change in deep-seated attitudes and beliefs, these media may nevertheless be used effectively to bring about a more hopeful and objective attitude in the community at large. This is particularly the case with television, because of its semi-personal nature, the great number of people it reaches, and its influence with persons of below-average education and intelligence who generally find it difficult to visualize many concepts presented by the spoken or written word.

To overcome programming difficulties inherent in telecasting a film, interview or panel discussion on cancer, the Anti-Cancer Council of Victoria has produced a 60-second educational 'commercial' presenting the "seven warning signs" in animated form. This was made freely available to all television stations in Victoria, and two years after its release is still being televised regularly; it is screened without charge by the stations concerned as a community service. The 'commercial' has also been screened by television stations in some other states.

The Australian Broadcasting Commission, a federal statutory body, has co-operated in cancer education at a national level, particularly by televising in all states two Victorian-produced films concerned with cancer diagnosis, treatment and cure: "Another Day" and "You are not alone".

Radio, despite the popularity of television, remains an important medium, particularly in country areas. In Tasmania, a lecturer of the State Cancer Committee broadcasts a weekly health programme in which aspects of cancer control are regularly discussed. A series of recorded talks and two dramatised programmes specially prepared for broadcasting have been used extensively by Victorian stations, and the state cancer organizations in Queensland and New South Wales have also utilised the medium of radio.

The Australian press plays a significant part in promoting education on cancer. The country and suburban press in particular has shown a lively interest and responsibility, and in those states where an active education campaign is under way the district papers as a rule carry full and accurate reports of local meetings. In addition many papers reprint short articles on cancer supplied by the state health authorities or Cancer Councils.

Educational programmes have been influenced by public opinion surveys carried out in Brisbane, Melbourne and Perth, which have provided information about attitudes to the disease and about prevailing areas of misconception and inadequate knowledge.

Canada

The most distinctive feature of public education about cancer in Canada is the pre-eminent role of the Canadian Cancer Society, formed in 1938. Other agencies which play lesser roles are the various government Departments of Public Health, the Canadian Medical Association and the educational authorities responsible for health teaching in schools.

The original, and for some time, almost the sole objective of the Canadian Society's educational programme was to promote early diagnosis and early treatment of cancer. On the basis of evidence available at that time it seemed reasonable to believe that a significant reduction in cancer mortality might be achieved by persuading people to watch for the first manifestations of malignant disease

and then go quickly to their doctor. Moreover, physicians treating cancer were impressed by the relatively large number of patients who, when first seen, had advanced or extensive disease and who would admit delay in seeking medical attention. It seemed logical to assume that many of the deaths among this group might be prevented if earlier diagnoses could be achieved. Based on these assumptions, the Society proclaimed widely "The Seven Danger Signals of Cancer" and urged those observing them to see their doctor without delay.

Within a few years it became apparent that the "Danger Signals" programme was less effective than had been anticipated. Many cancer patients still procrastinated instead of seeking prompt medical care. Efforts were redoubled to spread more widely and emphasize more strongly the gospel of early diagnosis but the gains were less dramatic than had been hoped for.

To determine the effectiveness of its programme, the Society conducted a number of surveys of public opinion about cancer. Each survey was carried out by an independent professional organization in order to avoid the possibility of bias and to ensure proper sampling. The surveys of women's opinions were carried out in 1954 and in 1960 and the survey of men's opinions was conducted in 1961. Although the survey showed that there had been an increase in knowledge about cancer, it was noted that 75% of women and 50% of men gave fear as the main reason for delay in seeking treatment for cancer.

Cancerphobia now became a prime target of the Society's educational programme. To attack this problem, efforts were made to de-emphasize the penalties for delay and, instead, to stress the benefits of early diagnosis. Survival-rates were presented in their most optimistic form; mortality figures were not mentioned. In all discussions of cancer, emphasis was placed on the positive rather than the negative aspects of the subject. Attention was focussed on the fact that many patients with cancer can be cured and that all patients with cancer can be helped — even those with types of disease for which modern treatment does not yet promise a cure.

In recent years attempts have been made to devise a more sophisticated approach to the problem of cancerphobia. The objective now is to foster the development of a rational attitude towards cancer and in so doing to eliminate the irrational fear of cancer. If people can be taught to face up to cancer calmly and sensibly, to see the disease in fair perspective in relation to other hazards which threaten us all, to reduce the emotional charge associated with the word "cancer" — then, and, only then, can they be expected to participate intelligently in plans for its prevention and control.

It is also important that doctors, nurses, health-educators and Cancer Society workers should themselves try to come to grips with the problem of cancerphobia. If these people can work out for themselves a sensible understanding of cancer — if they can talk about it calmly and unemotionally — if they can accept without panic the fact that they themselves might develop cancer — then shall they be in a position to influence others and to dispel fear.

There are many indications that efforts along these lines have borne fruit. Investigations and surveys have shown that more patients are reporting with their disease at an early stage; more people are familiar with the early signs of cancer; irrational fear of cancer seems to be less prevalent. But despite these achievements the survival statistics improved less rapidly than had been hoped,

so attention was directed to methods of early detection by periodic health examinations and by self-examination of the female breast. The Canadian Cancer Society still promotes such health checks, but is careful not to exaggerate their effectiveness and suggests that doctors should explain to their patients the limitations of these procedures.

In recent years the emphasis has shifted to cancer prevention, in which lies the greatest hope for the future. The two most obvious examples — the reduction of cigarette smoking and the discovery of premalignant lesions of the uterine cervix by mass cytological screening — have become a major preoccupation of the Society's programme.

The philosophy and objectives of the Society's education policy are largely determined by the National Education Committee which is also responsible for most pamphlets, booklets, films and filmstrips. In actual fact, most of the major movies and some of the pamphlets are Canadian adaptations of material produced by the American Cancer Society. Occasionally movies from other countries, particularly Great Britain, have also been used to advantage here.

Each of the ten Provincial Divisions of the Canadian Cancer Society has its own Education Committee which selects various aspects of the National Education programme for special emphasis, maintains liaison with the provincial medical society and educational authorities and which may develop educational material, including films, for use within that province or elsewhere.

Within each province are a large number of units through which actual contact with the citizens is achieved. All units have an Education Committee which plans and carries out a continuous educational programme using volunteer workers. The objective is to reach all the people (a) through news media, television, radio and movies (b) in their homes by house-to-house visits and home meetings (c) in schools and colleges (d) at their place of work — factories, offices, lumber camps, civil service departments, etc., (e) wherever people meet in groups, e. g. fraternal organizations, church societies, conventions, fairs, etc.

A special effort is made to maintain good relations with the Press. Whenever possible, a representative of the Press is appointed to the Education Committee. News releases are prepared at National and Divisional Cancer Society offices and distributed through units to local newspapers. Press coverage is always sought for major educational efforts such as cancer forums, public showings of cancer movies, cancer educational conferences, etc.

The initiation of a Cancer Education programme in the schools begins with securing an endorsation from the Provincial Department of Education. With this approval unit education committees can approach local Boards of Education, school principals and teachers. The objective is to encourage the inclusion of information about cancer in the regular Health and Science classes and to offer help in this work by providing literature and visual aids. Special effort is directed to the problem of cigarette smoking — whenever opportunity presents the Cancer Society will arrange for a well-qualified physician to meet and talk with students on this subject and to participate in panel discussions or debates. The Cancer Society has also sponsored essay contests in many areas, which have served to direct attention and thought to the relationship of smoking and lung cancer. In this connection surveys carried out by the Canadian Cancer Society have shown that many children begin to smoke cigarettes as early as grade V (10—12 years).

Hence it is now felt that efforts to discourage smoking should be started in grade IV and continued year by year at a progressively increasing level of sophistication throughout primary and secondary schools.

Parent-Teacher Associations are highly developed in Canada. Through such organisations parents can be told the facts of the smoking and health problem and their co-operation solicited in the campaign to protect their children from this hazard.

Chile

In 1938, doctors from the Instituto del Radium in Santiago and prominent personalities of the community founded the Chilean League Against Cancer. Among the declaration of principles of the League it was stated:

".... to penetrate public conscience through a permanent propaganda at all social levels with the knowledge of the dangers of cancer and the methods of restoring health .... to point out to the public the means to prevent cancer and offer them the known methods of treatment ..."

The League, soon after its foundation, started a programme on public education which included: periodical lectures through radio and comprehensive articles in the most important newspapers and magazines; short lectures to school teachers, students of the higher grades, medical students, nurses, social workers, etc. At the end of the lectures, small booklets with the danger signs and on specific types of cancer, were distributed; sometimes, through the courtesy of the American Embassy, a motion picture was shown.

The League also sponsored medical congresses and meetings in several of the main cities in the Country which lasted approximately three to seven days. During this period of time a massive educational campaign for the public was done through the usual channels of public information. Unions were approached, women were gathered together, schools were visited. People were encouraged to support the League or to form their own local leagues.

The philosophy of this programme was based on the principles that there are certain symptoms and signs that may be caused by cancer, that the disease is curable when it is treated in time and that the adults should have a medical examination at least once every year.

The League continued working with a certain amount of efficiency until 1957. Since then, practically speaking, the only public education about cancer have been our cancer congresses, where again activity is developed through the radio and the newspapers.

The League obtains its funds partly from private institutions and individuals and mostly from government aid, but its total yearly income is very meagre; in 1964 it was less than 4.000 dollars.

In 1954, thanks to the generosity of a Chilean lady living in Europe, a new cancer institute was created, the "Instituto de Oncología, Fundación Arturo López Pérez". This institute, which is concerned with detection, diagnosis, treatment and research about cancer, is now studying a public educational programme to be conducted in an area of Santiago, the capital city.

There has been no serious investigation of the effectiveness of the public educational campaign about cancer, and nothing is known with certainty about the reaction of the population to the information given. On the other hand, we do not know either what the people think about cancer, or if the methods employed to reach them have established some communication with them. On the contrary, indirect evidence points to the fact that

very little, if anything, has been accomplished and that the great mass of the population did not receive the information or were not motivated by it:

a) In ten years, less than 10.000 women have sought a medical examination or a vaginal smear test at the Female Detection Clinic in Santiago.

b) The readily detectable cancers such as uterus, breast, skin, etc., still come to us in advanced stages of their disease.

It is true that this is not always the case with the more educated patients, who ask more frequently for vaginal smears and, their lesions, as a whole, are not as advanced as in the great bulk of the population.

If this presents a rather gloomy view of what has been achieved, it has to be borne in mind that, in a country with serious economic problems, the national health authorities are forced to give priority in their budgetary arrangements to the control of diseases and conditions that are easily prevented or ameliorated by relatively simple hygiene measures (e. g. tuberculosis and the diseases of infancy that spring from poverty and inadequate living standards). Despite the lack of a concerted educational effort aimed at the early diagnosis and prevention of cancer, it cannot be said that the government has been totally indifferent to the problem. The prerequisite of any educational programme — the availability of adequate treatment facilities — has been met by the development throughout the country of cancer treatment centres and the establishment of a nation-wide cancer registry.

Denmark

This work has, for a number of years, been based solely on educational meetings and folders which gave data on the symptoms of cancer and appealed to the public to seek medical advice in every case where it was thought that any of these symptoms were evident. However, it was noted in these folders, so as to avoid creating unnecessary fear, that only in a minority of cases did these symptoms actually indicate cancer, but that it would not, of course, do any harm to have other less serious illness treated and cured.

The information meetings are primarily arranged by the local units of the Society, of which there are 190 distributed over the entire country. Meetings are often arranged in co-operation with other societies, especially women's groups and women's trade unions.

At the meetings, where there is always free admission, folders and brochures are distributed — also without charge — and there are opportunities for members of the audience to join the Society, just as everyone is given opportunity, at every meeting, to ask questions of the lecturer.

The lecturer may be a local doctor who can get information for the preparation of his lecture from the headquarters of the Society. If the meeting is held as part of a national campaign, the headquarters of the Society can supply complete lecture manuscripts which may be used in their entirety or rewritten by the lecturing physician in his own words.

Practically speaking, the lectures are always about a specific form of cancer (e. g., cancer of the uterus) and only those types of cancer where there is hope of successful treatment after an early diagnosis. The lecture often ends with a few remarks about cancer in general and the importance of early treatment. All meetings are open to both men and women.

As in the lectures, the information folders are aimed at specific forms of cancer and they are written by specialists in the specific fields they treat. All of the folders contain descriptions of the common danger signals one should be on the watch for.

It has not been found to be expedient to run a continuous information campaign. It is as if the public becomes tired of and uninterested in the propaganda while, in contrast, the periodic campaigns create significant interest, not only for the specific type of cancer being discussed, but also for other forms of cancer. In this manner, it is also much easier to interest the daily press.

Each effort within the information programme is planned very carefully. Contact is made with the various physician's and surgeon's societies which may be affected by the campaign, in order to secure their co-operation. Furthermore, an investigation is made to determine the possibilities for treating the patients which will be discovered as a result of the information programme and who will seek medical assistance and be referred to a specialist for examination and perhaps treatment.

Posters are also used, but this is an expensive form of advertising and the number of possible outdoor outlets are severely restricted in Denmark. Short advertising films and still slides are used in cinemas, as are the special films produced by the National Society and distributed on free loan to local units or organizations which apply for them.

With the growth of television, it has become increasingly difficult to attract audiences to meetings of any kind. It has therefore become necessary to seek a closer associatian with radio and television. However, broadcasting time is limited and there are no more than four radio lectures per year, including one on cancer in the regular series "The Radio Doctor". Television is used on the occasion of the annual Cancer Day and whenever there is news of advances in the cancer field at home or abroad.

There are many individual examples of the importance of the information programme's significance in the early treatment and curing of cancer, but a statistical analysis, as such, was first made in 1964, when the Cancer Register established and run by the Cancer Society investigated the results of a campaign instituted by the Society in the period 1951—54 for self-examination of the breast. The result was an improvement in the survival-rate during nine years and the Society is now considering a new campaign of the same character.

One handicap within cancer information work exists in Denmark. It is extremly seldom that a physician tells his patient that he has cancer. If he is cured, no-one hears of it, but if he dies, everyone knows that it was cancer. This gives the population the impression that the chances of a successful cure are less than they are in reality. A little more optimism could possibly bring even more to an early treatment.

France

There is in France a national organization responsible for general health education of the public, but since the Ligue National Française contre le Cancer (L.N.F.) was formed earlier and included most of the country's cancer specialists, most education of the public concerning cancer has remained in the hands of the L.N.F. Within the Ligue National there is a regional organization based on administrative "départements". Each departmental committee organizes its own propaganda programme with the help of the Social Security organization of the region.

Every year since 1950, the L.N.F. has conducted an annual campaign lasting for a week, culminating in a national fund-raising drive. Propaganda against cancer is undertaken mainly in the two months prior to the fund-raising campaign and reaches its peak during the "Cancer Week". Pamphlets giving a wide range of information about cancer and its treatment are available for distribution, and posters commissioned by the L.N.F. from artists of high quality are sent to regional committees for display during "Cancer Week".

Public meetings on cancer are arranged from time to time, usually comprising a 30-minute lecture by a doctor (preferably a specialist in cancer) and the showing of films. The subject of the lecture is fairly general, dealing with the frequency of various forms of cancer, its insidious onset, the first signs of warning, the greater curability of cases detected early, etc. The provision of suitable films for such meetings has proved extremely difficult. Some have presented an oversimplified picture of reasonable and unreasonable behaviour and so have been unconvincing. The most effective, it seems, have been short films of interviews with cured patients and one which shows the working of a cancer hospital, the simplicity of modern treatments and medical advice, and information about research in progress.

Television and radio are also used, though almost exclusively during "Cancer Week". The best T.V. sequences have been those filmed in hospitals, with doctors and patients interviewed in turn, including people who have been cured of cancer many years ago. Newspapers also participate in "Cancer Week" and publish articles by prominent cancer specialists.

But more efficient than the general propaganda directed indiscriminately is that directed to special groups, and particularly to young boys and girls about to leave school (16—18 years old). Special lectures are given by doctors to these young people, but information is also provided by the school-teachers themselves in the natural sciences curriculum.

For this purpose, the L.N.F. has prepared and published a sample lesson, which is constantly kept up-to-date.

However, the greatest effort has to be concentrated on the education of doctors themselves if they are to enable their patients to obtain the maximum benefit from the campaign of public education.

Netherlands

In the Netherlands, the so-called Cross societies (secular, protestant and catholic organizations) have, since the early 1920s, gradually acquired responsibility for public health education. However, over the years other organizations devoted to fighting one or other of the major diseases have been formed. One of these is the Netherlands Cancer Society, which is concerned with all aspects of the fight against cancer. A central institute now exists to coordinate the various health education programmes, and one of the participating bureaux is the Bureau for Cancer Registration and Education, which is the focal point of the cancer education programme in the Netherlands and also, since 1964, of the campaign against cigarette smoking.

The programme of the Bureau has been based on the possibilities for the early detection of cancer. There have been pilot schemes for the detection of cervical cancer by Pap smears, but no major effort has so far been directed at forms of the disease other than lung cancer. In the Netherlands, there is agreement on the point that public education should precede nation-wide screening programmes, with the aim of increasing public knowledge to the point where early diagnosis will raise the overall survival-rate for cancers to 50 per cent. Public education has to go hand-in-hand with professional education, since not all doctors are yet convinced of the advantages of public education. Their opinion is to some extent a reflection of their own pessimistic views of cancer prognosis.

Since the major difference between survival-rates for men and women in the Netherlands (23 % against 37 %) is accounted for by lung cancer deaths, the major effort of the Bureau has been directed into the campaign against smoking. Less effort has been devoted to cervical cytology, since deaths from cervical cancer account for only 3% of female cancer deaths in Holland.

The anti-smoking campaign has been organized by the Bureau, but financed by the government, which has taken a positive stand in several ways, including the imposition of an additional tax of 25% on cigarettes. The initial government grant for public education (200,000 florins = $ 56,000 U.S.) was raised in 1965 to 350,000 florins ($ 98,000 U.S.), a powerful public demonstration of how seriously the government regards the problem. There has been a concentrated educational effort throughout all schools, in all teacher-training colleges, among parents and the adult population generally, and among all sections of the medical profession. Special literature has been distributed, aimed at particular age-groups and sections of the community, and there has been invaluable support from the press, radio and television. Some results have already been achieved: in 1964 cigarette consumption decreased by 20% in the Netherlands.

A bi-annual periodical produced by the Cancer Society is distributed to its 210,000 members, informing them of achievements in treatment and research. A bulletin is also being produced for the regular supply of information to the press, and a booklet, "Facts About Cancer", is to have a first public distribution of 260,000 in 1965. Public meetings are also arranged at which physicians and district nurses give lectures on cancer, similar to those given in the U.K. (Manchester scheme) and in Denmark.

United Kingdom

"We are convinced that education aiming at a truer understanding of cancer and the methods for early detection can do nothing but good. Unreasonable fear of cancer is caused by ignorance, not by knowledge." So ran the comment of an official committee appointed to consider the future of health education in Great Britain, whose report was published in 1964. It is remarkable that such a statement need have been made at all, but the painful fact is that no national scheme of public education about cancer exists in Britain, although the Ministry of Health has since 1952 encouraged county and city local governments to promote health education about cancer in their own localities. Largely because of the initiative of voluntary agencies, cancer education has been developed in several parts of the country, with notable centres of activity in York, Oxford, Cardiff and the Liverpool and Manchester regions. Of these the then Manchester Committee on Cancer was in 1952 the first to launch a large-scale project of cancer education, and is now the most extensive, serving an area with a population in excess of 4,000,000. There are minor differences between the methods and media used in the five regions, but in broad terms a description of the philosophy and methods of the Manchester Regional Committee on Cancer is representative of such cancer education as is being undertaken in Britain.

The aims of the Manchester project are based on the results of special baseline studies, conducted before the scheme began, into public attitudes to and beliefs about cancer and into the reasons why patients with disquieting symptoms may defer seeking medical advice. In broad terms they are:

1. To disseminate authoritative information about cancer, with an emphasis on the less well-known reassuring facts.

2. To allay needless fears, correct mistaken beliefs, and to promote more confidence in the value of early treatment.

3. To educate the public about preventive measures

From the beginning the Committee has been fortunate in having the experience of pioneers in the field, such as the American and Canadian Cancer Societies, to draw on; but it was also guided by evidence that person-to-person communications, especially where opportunity is allowed for questions and free discussion, are the most effective in changing attitudes. It therefore attempts to achieve person-to-person contact with a large proportion of the population by means of a three-point approach; to people where they meet, where they learn and where they work. Firstly it supplies speakers — nearly all of them doctors concerned in the treatment of cancer — free of charge to voluntary groups and societies of all kinds. Secondly, the committee supplies speakers and visual aids and other background materials to schools and colleges, both to give young people a greater understanding of the nature of cancer, so that they may be armed against the influence of prejudices and mistaken beliefs about cancer which they will encounter among their elders, and to instruct them about the hazards of cigarette smoking. Thirdly, people are reached at their places of work. Following the pattern set by the Ontario Division of the Canadian Cancer Society, a mobile information service is provided for business and industry. A nurse, who is also a trained schoolteacher, is employed as full-time lecturer with special responsibility for the business and industry programme.

Apart from short reports in the local press which bring the main points of talks to a wider audience, the Committee at present uses little printed matter. This should not be taken to imply a criticism of the use of printed matter *per se*. It does, however, accept research findings that the effect of printed material compares unfavourably with other more personal methods of influencing behaviour and therefore feels that its limited budget can more profitably be expended on other outlets.

Such statistics as it quotes are connected with cure, rather than death; with the encouraging rewards of early treatment, rather than the dangers of delay. Every attempt is made to maintain a positive, health-orientated approach, and as far as possible to avoid fostering a preoccupation with disease. In view of the present climate of opinion regarding cancer in Britain, the Committee has not felt able to publicise the "Danger Signals of Cancer" that have been a key factor in cancer education in other countries. Although in person-to-person teaching, "Warning Signs" are always described, these are invariably discussed as signs of ill-health which call for prompt medical advice, rather than as symptoms of cancer.

If one particular approach could be said to colour the Committee's messages to the general public, it is that people are addressed not so much as potential victims ("This can happen to you"), but as potential helpers of friends and relatives who may be afflicted. Studies suggest that this is a more tolerable role for the audience, and it may be that acceptance of the message (which, since it concerns cancer, must in some degree arouse anxiety) is thereby made less difficult for the individual.

Manifestly any attempt to change for the better public opinion about cancer must have the full support of doctors and nurses. Limited enquiries among doctors and medical students, and a larger, intensive study among nurses have revealed a marked tendency towards unwarranted despondency about cancer. The Committee's programme therefore includes regular lectures to professional medical organizations and to nurses undergoing initial and in-service training at a number of local centres. The main aim of these talks is to impress on medical professionals the excellent results to be gained by the early treatment of cancer of certain sites, and to gain not only their acquiescence but also their active support in educating the public about cancer.

Evaluation of the results and other investigations are planned as an integral part of the educational programme, so that educators in the field may identify problems worthy of deeper study, while research findings are fed back into the educational programme as a means of refining techniques or organization. It is the constant interchange of ideas and hard facts between practitioners and researchers that is vital to the continuing vigour and viability of public education about cancer.

U.S.A.

Frank public discussion about cancer leads to more knowledge and better understanding of the disease. As gloomy fatalism is replaced by a life-preserving philosophy, attitudes and motivation change and lead to more reasoned and appropriate behaviour. This has been the view of the American Cancer Society since 1937 when it began its first national systematic efforts to communicate with the public. While there is still some mindless panic about cancer, the Society believes that the disease today is most often regarded realistically: a serious threat but free of much of its age-old aura of terror and mystery.

The Society believes in a broad communications approach to motivate a population now close to 200 million. People must be reached where they live or work; where they study, worship or relax; when they read newspapers, watch television, listen to radio or go to meetings. Mass communications media are most effective against cancer when joined with or accompanying an immediate, person-to-person approach in which the individual has the chance to ask questions, to express his own anxieties, present doubts and fears openly. In cancer the advice of a respected friend or acquaintance — with or without special medical training — can play a vital role.

The intention has been: (1) to build understanding and support for the broad attack on cancer (by the public, government agencies, and the medical profession at large); and (2) to teach individuals what they can do to protect themselves against the disease.

The tone of the Society's messages to the public is vigorous, optimistic, and often even evangelistic. Waging a battle in the market place of ideas with the other persistent claimants for the public ear, the Society uses advertisements contributed by the nation's many magazines; millions of copies of publications ranging from a cartoon booklet to relatively complex brochures; motion pictures, more than 25 of which are now in circulation; parades and meetings; and, the communications media themselves.

The intent in all these cases is to involve people in action to protect themselves; to reassure the frightened and to stimulate the indifferent; to persuade people to support cancer control activity, both as volunteer workers and as financial contributors.

"The earlier the diagnosis, the better" has been the Society's long-time message in cancer control, and will continue to be. A key element in this message has been the statistical observation that before World War II, only one-in-five of those with cancer was saved, whereas progress has been made since then. Gradual improvement followed, climbing to a ratio of one-in-four — and then (circa 1956) — to one-in-three. This figure still stands, although (if all patients were diagnosed and treated at as early a stage as possible) it could be reduced to on-in-two.

Statistical facts are informative; they are productive — and they are not motivational enough. People are more interested in other people than in statistics — people believe people. For this reason, the American Cancer Society does much of its education through speakers and through stories and pictures of individuals who have — at this time, at this place, in this way, with these results — been cured of cancer.

Perhaps the most constructive force in the United States has been the physician — a key figure in health education. The doctor's willingness to speak about cancer at meetings, to permit himself to be quoted by name in newspapers, to participate in television programs about the disease, has been an essential element in counteracting fear. In exchanges of patient and doctor at public meetings where questions may be raised and calmly answered, in newspaper columns by doctor-journalists, the work of reassurance and persuasion goes on. Most important, if behavior is to be changed, is for the individual to have the opportunity to express candidly his suspicions and worries and fears. These can be answered effectively by wise physicians.

With its more than 3,000 Units organized into 58 Divisions, the American Cancer Society has placed strong reliance on the notion of "association". Distribution of printed materials, exhibition of films, the spread of the anti-cancer message — all of these activities are predicated on the assumption that a significant fraction of the people will, in fact, come together to work for the common good. With only a skeleton of paid staff, the Society could never manage to bring its message home to a huge nation, the secret lies in the volunteer whether lay or professional.

The volunteer in the local community is typically a housewife; a woman who finds that a few hours a month of work for the American Cancer Society provide satisfaction and pleasure. In such a milieu the volunteer usually gains something; self-confidence and a broadened circle of friends. Not a few of the volunteers have themselves been cured of cancer and so have special motivation. Reasons for volunteering are often complex, a sound mixture of public service and self-interest; whatever the reasons, the impact on cancer control has been great. A major problem is equipping this volunteer so she may be a reliable source of information. In one of its recent projects the Society has developed a training kit of materials under the heading "Tell Your Neighbor" to illustrate content and show procedure for spreading information that may save lives from cancer.

The American Cancer Society has conducted a number of programs aimed at detection and treatment of cancer in certain body-sites. The most successful — as indicated above — has dealt with cancer of the uterus, with emphasis in recent years on the Pap test (cytology).

Brilliantly organized programs in such cities as Toledo, Philadelphia, Memphis, San Diego, Cleveland have brought many millions of women to have the test — however, it is striking that despite intensive work, not more than 70 per cent of wom-

en have had cytology in any urban area. Nevertheless, despite many years of intensive education, a recent study has shown that only half the women in America said they had had a Pap test.

Other site programs have concentrated on self-examination of the female breast and, more recently, on the desirability of regular proctosigmoidoscopic examination to combat cancer of the colon/rectum.

The causal link between cigarettes and lung cancer has absorbed much of the Society's interest. The Society believes (and is supported by surveys) that despite gloomy predictions that teen-agers would not be influenced by sensible warnings about risks far in the future, there has been some success in deterring young people from beginning to smoke. Factors in this include probably: 1. the report to the Surgeon General of the United States on *Smoking and Health* and other widely publicized documents; 2. the public's increasing realization that cigarette smoking is a risk; and 3. the reasonable approach which the Society has developed within schools. In spite of encouraging results in persuading youngsters to put off beginning to smoke, there is little evidence that those who have already started the habit have been influenced

A most important development has been the formation of the National Interagency Council on Smoking and Health, in which some eighteen health, educational, and governmental organizations have united. The Council led the fight in Congress for legislation requiring health warnings on cigarette packages, which was passed, and for similar warnings on advertising, which was defeated. Stronger legislation is hoped for in the future. Leading in the formation of the Council were the American Heart Association, the National Tuberculosis Association, the United States Public Health Service, the American Public Health Association and the Cancer Society.

The Society tries to evelute programs under way and afterwards. It is also currently planning a large study of public attitudes to, and behaviour in the face of, cancer.

U.S.S.R.

One of the main tasks of health education on cancer control in the Soviet Union is to interpret to the public the ways and possibilities of cancer prevention through timely treatment and the cure of precancerous conditions. The methods and content of cancer education were worked out on the basis of epidemiological data for the various regions of the U.S.S.R. and on studies of what people thought and knew about the possibilities of prevention.

Certain precancerous disorders — usually associated with unhealthy practices or harmful habits of long standing — were found to be particularly prevalent in certain areas of the vast territory of the U.S.S.R., e.g. leukoplakia of the buccal cavity in the Central Asian Republics, associated with the chewing of *nass* (a mixture of tobacco, ash and lime). However, a survey of the health behaviour of over 20,000 people revealed that only a small number were aware of the preventive measures available to them and how to protect themselves from harmful influences in the environment. The least well-informed were in remote rural communities.

Programmes aimed at timely detection and treatment of precancerous diseases conducted on the national level are being implemented in the country through regular and general mass and individual prophyplactic screening of the whole population, through the establishment of specialized "examination rooms" at outpatient health establishments, through the "dispensarization" of the public (constant medical follow-up), providing chronic patients with medical diet and accommodation at the over-night sanatoria owned by industrial enterprises, through a wide network of rest homes and sanatoria, etc. A study of the public's attitude towards cancer prevention showed that the people did not appreciate the subject enough: Those suffering from precancerous disorders were very apathetic about seeking a physician's advice and negative in observing it.

Our surveys and investigations showed that people suffering from pre-cancerous diseases did not make full use of all the existing facilities offered by the State free of charge, because they knew very little or nothing at all about real possibilities of preventing cancer by timely cure of the pre-cancerous states. The study showed also that people had very little understanding of the nature, causes and the development of pre-cancerous diseases. Most of the people interviewed, especially those in some regions of Moldavia, the Ukraine, the Central Asian and Transcaucasian Republics, did not appreciate, for example, the significance of health diet practices, regularity of meal times, in particular. Even more did not consider it harmful to take very hot tea and food regularly; quite a number of the local population did not think excessive exposure to sunlight harmful for the skin, and did not protect their faces from the hot southern sun. They also knew little about cancerogenic effects of smoking, or chewing *nass*; the women knew very little about the dangers of repeated abortions and were not aware of the possible aftereffects of their unwillingness to breast-feed their children on the appearance and development of pre-cancerous diseases of the breast.

In contrast to these examples of poor information, much wider knowledge on the part of the public on the ways of cancer prevention was registered in the regions where wide-scale sound health education programmes, scientifically and methodologically based, had been conducted (e. g. in Moscow, the city of Perm, and others).

Health education in the field of cancer prevention based on such studies is carried out in the U.S.S.R. in the following ways:

1. Explanation of the significance of timely cure of precancerous diseases as a practical way of preventing cancer; directed at the adult population, mostly among chronic patients.

2. Dissemination of health knowledge conducive to the prevention of the conditions which, if they progress, may in time offer fertile ground for cancer to arise. Directed at apparently healthy people of all ages.

The methods used in conveying information that will help to prevent the development of cancer are governed by the principle that it is most desirable to avoid iatrogenic reactions from the public. The term "precancerous disease" is not used; stress is laid on the fact that chronic disease does not always lead to cancer and that prevention of cancer can be achieved by timely treatment and cure of a chronic condition.

The peculiarity of the educational method lies mainly in the following: many factors of the environment together with regular violations of health behaviour are treated not as an immediate cancer challenge, but as important in stimulating certain conditions that may, if they progress, contribute to the appearance of cancer.

Cancer education is a component of the overall public health programme in the U.S.S.R. Certain steps have been taken to put this into effect:

1. Handbooks have been published, with guides to methods of cancer education, lecturers' kits with texts and charts (e. g. on breast self-examination and the harmful effects of smoking), slides, filmstrips and special educational instructions for those areas of the country where certain precancerous conditions are prevalent.

2. New films for the general public have been produced.

3. Booklets, pamphlets and leaflets are produced for the general public; also posters, wallcharts, displays and material for the press.

4. Special T.V. and radio programmes are broadcast, as well as items for inclusion in regular magazine programmes. The Central Institute for Research in Health Education prepares material for use by local T.V. and radio stations.

5. Training in the methodology of health education is given to physicians at Institutes for postgraduate instruction. Lectures are given to the general public by cancer specialists. Volunteers, mostly members of the Red Cross and Red Crescent, give considerable assistance to professionals involved in the work of health education.

Author Index

Pages on which the names of authors are mentioned within the short textual sections are not included in the index. Each reference is to the main bibliographical entry at the end of each textual section.

UICC Publications

Kaposi's Sarcoma. S. Karger AG., Basle (Switzerland) — New York (1963).

Cancer of the urinary bladder. S. Karger AG., Basle (Switzerland) — New York (1963).

Prognosis of malignant tumours of the breast. S. Karger AG., Basle (Switzerland) — New York (1963).

The lymphoreticular tumours in Africa. S. Karger AG., Basle (Switzerland) — New York (1964).

Cellular control mechanisms and cancer. Elsevier Publishing Company, Amsterdam — London — New York (1964).

Illustrated Tumor Nomenclature. Springer-Verlag, Berlin — Heidelberg — New York (1965).